Also by Bob Greene

Get With the Program!

The Get With the Program! Daily Journal

Keep the Connection:
Choices for a Better Body and a Healthier Life

Make the Connection: 10 Steps to a Better Body—
and a Better Life

Great Food for Good Health

SIMON & SCHUSTER
New York   London   Toronto   Sydney   Singapore

Bob Greene

The Get With the Program!

GUIDE TO GOOD EATING

This publication contains the opinions and ideas of its author. It is intended to provide helpful and informative material on the subjects addressed in the publication. It is sold with the understanding that the author and publisher are not engaged in rendering medical, health, psychological, or any other kind of personal professional services in the book. If the reader requires personal medical, health, or other assistance or advice, a competent professional should be consulted.

The author and publisher specifically disclaim all responsibility for any liability, loss, or risk, personal or otherwise, that is incurred as a consequence, directly or indirectly, of the use and application of any of the contents of this book.

SIMON & SCHUSTER
Rockefeller Center
1230 Avenue of the Americas
New York, NY 10020

Copyright © 2003 by Bob Greene
All rights reserved,
including the right of reproduction
in whole or in part in any form.

SIMON & SCHUSTER and colophon are registered trademarks
of Simon & Schuster, Inc.

MAKE THE CONNECTION AND GET WITH THE PROGRAM
are registered trademarks of Harpo, Inc.

For information regarding special discounts for bulk purchases,
please contact Simon & Schuster Special Sales at 1-800-456-6798
or business@simonandschuster.com

Designed by Bonni Leon-Berman

Manufactured in the United States of America

10 9 8 7 6 5 4 3 2 1

Library of Congress Cataloging-in-Publication Data

ISBN 0-7432-4310-2

Acknowledgments

With special thanks to Daryn Eller, Wendy Little, and Donna James Robb for their contribution to this work.

Contents

Introduction   1

PART I   Committing to a Healthy Lifestyle   11

Attitude Check   14

Maximizing Your Metabolism   15

    1. Staying Hydrated   16

    2. Working Out Aerobically   18

    3. Eliminating Emotional Eating   21

    4. Strength Training   24

PART II   The Guide to Good Eating   27

Four Steps to Good Eating   29

    Step 1: Eat a Nutritious Breakfast   29

    Step 2: Set an Eating Cutoff Time   40

    Step 3: Redistribute Your Calories   49

    Step 4: Make Healthful Food Choices   56

Creating a Healthy Kitchen   75

Eight Great Choices   79

Where to Shop for Good Food   84

Tips for Making Healthful Choices   90

Dining Out—And Staying on the Program   95

Being Good—But Not Perfect   100

PART III Recipes   103

Breakfast   105

Soups   119

Salads, Small Plates, and Sandwiches   133

Entrées   161

Side Dishes   187

Desserts   201

Index   218

The Get With the Program!

GUIDE TO GOOD EATING

Introduction

AS FAR BACK AS I CAN REMEMBER, I've been interested in the connection between food and good health. Even at the tender age of nine, I'd read in the paper about the health hazards of nitrates, then lobby my parents to banish bacon from our table. Though I was just a kid when word about the harmful effects of pesticides hit the headlines, I took the news to heart and worried about the quality of the produce my family was eating. What about the news (which turned out not to be true) that margarine is better than butter? I pestered my mom until she finally bought a tub of it. Or that salt causes high blood pressure? I warned my dad about using the shaker so liberally.

I guess you could say I was kind of an alarmist kid, but as the self-appointed guardian of my family's well-being, I took nutrition news seriously. And I still do, though I've learned that not everything you read in the papers and hear on the news is good solid advice—or that just because friends are into a new eating fad, you should be, too. I've also learned that while the more the average person learns about nutrition, the better, the sheer amount of information out there can be confusing. People are perplexed by all that they read and hear about nutrition and weight loss. Whenever I have a speaking engagement, I'm often bombarded with a million questions about crazy diets, "revolutionary" new foods and supplements that supposedly melt off pounds. People will also ask me for sound nutritional advice: Should I limit the amount of carbohydrates I eat? How many fat grams should I allow myself each day? Should I be taking nutritional supplements?

Nutrition, relatively speaking, is a very young science. But although we don't yet know everything about how good nutrition can help us stay healthy and lose weight, we do know a few key things. Foremost is that eating moderate amounts of nutritious foods—in combination with exercising regularly—is the number one way to ensure our well-being and fight the accumulation of body fat. Eat sensibly and exercise. It's a relatively simple prescription—and we know it works.

We also know what doesn't work, particularly in regard to weight loss. Americans have been dieting since the early 1900s (if not before; however, it's the crash diets of the last forty years that have really given us a crash course in what to avoid. I hate the idea that a lot of people (and possibly even you) have tried to lose on many of these programs, perhaps even gaining more weight in the process of yo-yoing from one diet to another. But these programs have at least taught us that going to extremes is an impractical—and clearly inadequate—way to slim down. And looking at them, you can see why.

Learning from Past Mistakes

Take *The Doctor's Quick Weight Loss Diet,* which helped to kick off the whole very-low-carbohydrate, high-protein approach to weight loss. Published by Dr. Irwin Stillman in 1967, *The Doctor's Quick Weight Loss Diet* dictated that its followers survive mainly on cottage cheese, eggs, seafood, poultry, and meat; fruits, vegetables, and grain foods were virtually forbidden.

Twenty million dieters tried Stillman's plan. The next fad: Dr. Robert Atkins's 1972 *Dr. Atkins' Diet Revolution,* another highly touted low-carbohydrate plan. This one let you eat just about all of the fat you wanted (and was the precursor of the diet Atkins still promotes today). It was followed in 1978, by *The Complete Scarsdale Medical Diet,* also low-carbohydrate, high-protein, and another top contender for American dieters' dollars.

What was the appeal of these low-carbohydrate, high-protein diets? For one thing, they *seemed* to work—but at what cost? People lost weight on them because eating high doses of protein causes the body to eliminate a lot of water weight. However, a very high-protein diet can also strain the kidneys and the liver and create a substance known as ketones. Ketones suppress the appetite (another reason the dieters might have lost weight). They also make you feel dizzy, cause bad breath and gas, and may contribute to gout and heart and kidney diseases.

Another problem associated with low-carbohydrate, high-protein eating is that it makes it harder to exercise effectively. That has to do with glycogen, a form of carbohydrate stored in the muscle and liver, and a primary source of fuel for exercise. If you don't have much glycogen left (which can easily occur if you are existing on a low-carbohydrate diet), you're not going to be able to exercise to the best of your ability—or, as a result, burn very many calories. The depletion of glycogen stores is also what causes low-carbohydrate, high-protein dieters to lose so much water and exaggerates their weight loss: for each gram of glycogen you use for energy, you give up about two and a half times that in water. The loss of glycogen and water makes it virtually impossible to exercise effectively.

Most people who were on these diets in the 1960s and 1970s weren't aware of what was going on in their bodies as they skimped on carbohydrates and filled up on protein. But even if they *were* cognizant of the health risks (and it's hard *not* to be aware of unpleasant side effects such as gas and bad breath), what ultimately made most of them throw in the towel was the fact that these diets, which restrict beloved foods such as bread, rice, and pasta—not to mention fruits and vegetables—are just too hard to stay on. Emotionally and physically, they're cruel deprivation. Few people can live on almost all protein. Eventually they give up and gain back all the weight, usually very quickly.

A lot of people got wiser after these failures, but some just went on to more extreme measures. In 1981, an even more restrictive low-carb, high-protein plan called the Cambridge Diet was introduced, and it quickly became all the rage—with dire consequences. This novel diet ensured that nobody had to worry about making the right food choices anymore because it involved no food—you had to consume only a couple of protein-rich liquid meals a day, totaling a mere 320 calories. Not surprisingly, the FDA and U.S. Postal Service quickly clamped down on mail-order sales of the diet, but its creators found a way to sell it through other means. At least until disaster struck. Many people on the Cambridge Diet started having health problems ranging from upset stomach to gallbladder problems, and then, sadly, about thirty of the dieters died.

There are still plenty of liquid diets around today, and, in fact, the Cambridge Diet is back, albeit reformulated and reportedly safer. In the 1980s, many people tried the medically monitored Optifast diet. Again, they shed pounds, only to put them all back on again—and then some. Liquid diets, regardless of how conscientiously they're created, rarely work over the long term. Nothing about a liquid diet prepares you to deal with the real food challenges you face once you stop sipping your meals. And trust me, eventually you'll have to start eating real food again.

Later in the 1980s (and into the 1990s), fat became diet enemy number one. Suddenly carbs were in and fat was out in a big way. Now, there is some legitimate concern about having too much fat in the diet. A high fat intake—especially a high saturated and hydrogenated fat intake—is linked to a variety of maladies, including obesity, cancer, and heart disease. But we do need *some* fat in our diets—it's essential for certain physiological processes to take place and it plays a role in how satisfied we feel after a meal. When you eat fat, your body gets the message that its needs are met and signals your brain to tell you to stop eating.

But even more significant is the fact that fat makes food taste good. Eating needs to be enjoyable as well as fulfill your nutritional needs, and fat plays an important part in making food not just palatable but delicious. If you take away all the fat, you take away much of the pleasure. Who can stay on a diet like that for very long? A plan that includes healthy fats in moderation (while limiting or eliminating the unhealthy saturated and trans-fats ones) offers you a much better chance of success.

Given all that, it's not surprising that despite the rash of diets that preached cutting fat to rock-bottom levels and the wave of fat-free foods that came onto the market to make it easier, many people still struck out; the diets were just too rigid and boring. Quite a few dieters even gained weight because they ate massive quantities of fat-free foods, not realizing that while the foods might have been free of fat, they were still chock full of calories, mostly from sugar. Like the very-low-carbohydrate diets before them, many of these very-low-fat plans have fallen out of favor.

Just about the time that fat was being cut from diets left and right, another option became available: sophisticated and heavily marketed pharmaceuticals that promised to help people slim down dramatically. It seemed as though the prayers for a magic pill that would burn off fat had finally been answered. Of course these drugs didn't work like magic, and some of them even turned out to have serious side effects. Most notably was Fen-phen, a weight loss drug cocktail that had to be pulled from the market because it was found to cause heart valve abnormalities. Even when people who took the drugs suffered no adverse side effects, they usually gained back the weight they'd lost when they went off the pills. Like the liquid diets before them, drugs can help you slim down, but they can't teach you to eat right or make you exercise.

Unfortunately, some of these pills are still out there, and we are likely to see more come onto the market in the next few years.

But even as diets and drugs come and go, there is always something new to replace them. Anyone who wants to lose weight is still faced with a lot of enticing come-ons that can be hard to resist. Lately, it's been the promise of quick loss on (yes, they're back!) low-carbohydrate, high-protein diets. These new versions aren't as extreme as the ones from the 1960s and 1970s, but they're similar. Some of them let you eat all the meat, fat, and eggs you can stomach and claim that you'll be healthier for it. Never mind that this simply goes against reason (not to mention an extensive body of research). When all evidence points to the fact that a diet rich in fruits, vegetables, and whole grains lowers the risk of many diseases, including various cancers, and that a diet rich in animal foods increases the risk, it doesn't make sense to substitute steak for salad. Is it worth risking your health just to be thin? And temporarily thin at that?

The diet industry often asks you to suspend logic. Could taking a tablespoon of something called Dream Away before bed really help you shed pounds overnight with no effort on your part? Of course not, but the very idea that it might work can make even a rational person take leave of her senses. The fitness industry also plays into our hopes. You may know in your heart of hearts that a piece of exercise equipment can't help you lose something unbelievable like twenty-five pounds in fourteen days. Yet there they are on the TV, men and women with cut bodies, looking as if they're having more fun exercising on a cheap piece of equipment than they would picnicking in the South of France, and promising to change your life. For many people, common sense be damned—it's hard not to buy into the dream.

An Approach to Good Health and Weight Loss You Can Trust

It's easy to knock the people in the diet and fitness industries who have led consumers down the wrong path. But the failures of all these diets and exercise gizmos bring us full circle to where we started: nothing works better than eating healthy foods in reasonable portions and exercising. That's what worked in 1960, and it's what works now. These days, though, we have significantly more information about the process of weight loss to guide us. We have a better understanding of how the body responds to food and exercise and greater knowledge about how big a role emotional eating and metabolism play in the whole equation. So while moderate eating and regular exercise are still the basic prescription for good health and weight loss, we can now also supplement them with other strategies that increase the likelihood of success.

In *Get With the Program!* I covered the first steps you need to take in order to lose weight: making a commitment to yourself, getting a grip on emotional eating, and becoming stronger and healthier through exercise. This companion book *The Get With the Program! Guide to Good Eating,* builds on those steps by giving you nutrition information that will show you how to choose good-quality food in reasonable quantities and how to reach your weight loss and fitness goals: by eating breakfast, having a cutoff time for eating, and redistributing your calories throughout the day.

Most weight loss programs start by addressing food, but I addressed it only briefly in *Get With the Program!* because I believe that first adopting positive behaviors such as exercising and dealing with emotional issues makes it easier to change your eating habits. It's also very important to rev up your metabolism with exercise *before* you start cutting calories. Cutting calories slows down your metabolism, but if you're already exercising, your metabolism will resist the slowdown and stay strong. If you aren't exercising yet (and by exercising I mean engaging in aerobic workouts and strength training), I suggest that you go back to *Get With the Program!* for guidance on how to get moving, or check out the recap in Part I of this book to "move" you in the right direction. Then, when you feel you're ready, begin taking steps toward more healthful eating.

There are plenty of misconceptions out there about what constitutes a healthy diet. We all hear a lot about nutrition, but often the information is misleading or even downright inaccurate. This book is devoted to setting the record straight and helping you make the right choices. It will help you lose weight. It's important, though, to keep weight loss in perspective. You may dream of being supermodel thin, but if it's not in your genetic makeup, you never will be. Nor should you *want* to be. This program is geared toward helping you realize your potential, and that means helping you become stronger and healthier. That may include losing a substantial amount of weight, or it may not. What's most important is that you find the courage to make the meaningful changes in your life. This will allow you to feel good both physically and emotionally as you reach the weight that is correct for your body type.

One thing I know for sure is that by following this sensible plan based on moderate eating and exercise, you will reach your goals. You may not reach them as quickly as you'd like—almost nobody does—but you will reach them. I'm not going to throw anything crazy at you, and I'm confident that you can handle all the steps to good eating that you will encounter in this book. That's because I'm not asking you to change your life overnight; that simply doesn't work. For change to really take effect, it has to be gradual. Quick fixes are seductive, but doing things the *right* way requires more time and quite a bit of patience. But it's worth it. You'll get the best results if you take it slowly, waiting until you master one step before moving onto the next.

What Lies Ahead

The Get With the Program! Guide to Good Eating is divided up into three main parts. In Part I, I go over the core principles that were described in *Get With the Program!* If you've read that book, this is a perfect opportunity for you to refresh your memory and check up on how you're doing. You may even want to renew your commitment to yourself by re-signing the "Contract with Myself" that was included in *Get with the Program!* If you're unfamiliar with the earlier book, Part I in this book will familiarize you with the behaviors that were integral to that program: increasing your water consumption, exercising aerobically, getting a handle on your emotional eating, and performing strength training exercises.

In Part II, I'll talk about why eating breakfast matters (I think you'll be surprised at how much it does) and why you need to cut out late-night eating. I'll also go over the importance of distributing your calories properly throughout the day and give you a quick course in nutrition to help you understand how different foods affect your body. After reading this, you'll better understand how to divvy up carbohydrates, fats, and proteins in your diet and how to make choices that will keep your energy—and your metabolism—revved up.

Finally, in Part III, you'll get some real specifics on how to eat well. Unless you've been living under a rock, you already know that you should eat more fruits, vegetables, and whole grains, but how can you actually incorporate them into your diet in an interesting and appealing way? Over the last few years, some foods have gotten a bad rap; I want to restore their reputation and tell you how they can be part of a healthy diet and even help you to lose weight. In Part III, you'll also learn how to dine out wisely and how to shop smart: when you're trying to drop pounds and eat healthfully, probably the most critical move you can make is simply to not put certain foods into your shopping cart.

In addition to all this, I am excited to bring you eighty truly wonderful recipes. These delicious dishes will quickly lay to rest the notion that healthy food is dull. For primitive men and women, the purpose of eating may have been simply to stay alive, but we are highly evolved beings! For us, eating is—or least should be—a pleasurable experience. It's part of our culture; many friendships and family relationships have been cemented over the sharing of good food. I hope that you won't let wanting to improve your health and lose weight exclude you from the joys of eating. It's time to take the guilt out of consuming good food, and these satisfying recipes do it beautifully. They'll help you enjoy yourself, safe in the knowledge that you are also eating intelligently.

I'm happy that you have made the choice to forgo get-thin-quick schemes in favor of *The Get With the Program! Guide to Good Eating*—it's your ticket to better physical health and well-being. In my years as an exercise physiologist, personal trainer, and author, I've had the good fortune to help many people reach their goals. You're next, so read on!

PART I

Committing to a **Healthy** **Lifestyle**

GETTING TO WHERE YOU WANT TO GO in life is a process. It takes time, commitment, and a series of accomplishments—some big, some small, but each important. Change is a progression, and each bit of progress you make gives you confidence to take on the next challenge. In *Get With the Program!* I introduced readers to several important behaviors that would powerfully alter their physical and emotional well-being. In case you missed *Get With the Program,* I'll quickly go over four of the most crucial of those behaviors in order to bring you up to date. If you read the previous book, this will serve as an excellent refresher course and help you stay on or get back on track.

Among these behaviors are two different types of exercise: aerobic workouts and strength training. You might wonder what exercise is doing in a guide to good eating, but I strongly believe that you can't separate the two. If you want to achieve wellness and weight loss, you have to do both: eat well *and* exercise. So why am I discussing exercise first? Because exercise can provide you with a powerful incentive to eat well. When you exercise, you really feel it if you're not properly fueled—it's hard to keep your energy up. Knowing that good nutrition will give you the strength and stamina you need to perform your workouts properly is going to make you want to eat well. You'll become much more conscious of what you're consuming. And exercise keeps your metabolism revved up, helping to counteract the metabolic slowdown that naturally occurs when you start cutting calories.

Exercise is an important part of the foundation upon which to build healthy eating habits. But another important—in fact, absolutely essential—component is your attitude. Your level of motivation and the way you think about your prospects of success are key. Just by reading this far, you're moving in the direction of change, but before you go any further it's time for an "attitude check."

Attitude Check

- **Reaching a certain size or weight won't necessarily make me happy.** Not unless you identify and deal with any underlying problems that have made weight an issue in your life.

- **There are no shortcuts to achieving what I want.** Dedication, commitment, and effort are needed to accomplish anything worthwhile.

- **Excuses ("I don't have time," "I'm too tired to exercise," "I've already blown it today, I'll start again tomorrow") just won't wash.** If you're ready to change, you're ready to stop making excuses.

- **Each improvement I make, not just pounds lost, is worth acknowledging and praising myself for.** Feeling better, sleeping better, feeling stronger, being less stressed, looking healthier—focus on these aspects of improvement, and you will keep your motivation up.

- **Setbacks are going to happen.** Setbacks are a natural and inevitable part of any progression and are no reason to throw in the towel. If you can overcome setbacks and reach your goals in spite of them, you have shown true strength of character. Ultimately, your sense of accomplishment will be that much greater.

- **Losing weight takes willpower.** As much as some people (those selling gimmicks under the guise "Weight Loss Made Easy") would like you to believe that you don't have to give up anything to slim down, the truth is that you do. Your commitment to your health and well-being will require some small sacrifices, but the return on your investment will be large.

• **Physical activity is nonnegotiable.** You have to move to improve.

• **I can love my family and friends and be a good employee and still take care of myself.** Get those close to you to support your program, and from this point on, consider your health and well-being sacred. Don't let your obligations to others interfere with your obligations to yourself.

If any of these statements makes you feel unsure about whether you can truly make a commitment to yourself right now, I recommend that you consider holding off until you feel ready to handle the challenge. And you will eventually feel ready—but you need to do it within your own time frame. If you do feel prepared for the challenges to come, keep reading. Some of what lies ahead may be tough, but it will be very rewarding.

Maximizing Your Metabolism

Let's talk about your metabolism. You're going to be hearing a lot about metabolism throughout this book, because the rate at which you burn calories (that's the definition of metabolism) is critical to maintaining a healthy weight. And *increasing* your metabolic rate is critical to *losing* weight permanently. Everybody burns calories at his or her own individual rate; if you've always had a sluggish metabolism, you'll probably never get it to run at the same speed as that skinny girl's from high school (who turned up at the class reunion twenty years later looking just as skinny). But you *can* maximize your metabolism's potential so that it burns at its highest rate for the largest number of hours per day.

One thing we know about metabolism is that it changes throughout the day; it is slowest when you're sleeping (even though you're asleep, you still must burn calories to maintain your body's basic functions, such as breathing, heartbeat, and digestion). We also know that certain things you do can give your metabolism a boost. Eating is one of them. Exercise is another (although exercise raises your calorie-burning rate much more than eating). As soon as you begin exercising—whether doing aerobic exercise or strength training—your metabolism increases, and it continues to increase in direct proportion to the length and intensity of your workout. Best of all, the boost your metabolism gets from exercise can last for hours after you've stepped off the treadmill or put down the weights. But the really good news is that you can increase your metabolism 24 hours a day, 365 days a year with consistent exercise. This is how dramatic weight loss occurs.

In the pages that follow, you'll learn a lot more specifics about your metabolism and how you can change it. You already know that burning calories through exercise and eating fewer calories will help you lose weight. But metabolism is another and entirely separate piece of the puzzle. Boosting yours is the first order of business. Let's identify the four behaviors that make up the foundation of good eating and that will keep your metabolism running efficiently.

1. Staying Hydrated

> GOAL: Start drinking a minimum of 6 eight-ounce glasses of water
> a day, and work up to 9.

Since water has no calories, most people think it doesn't have anything to do with weight loss. But it does, and it's essential for good health. When you're dehydrated, your body's ability to perform virtually every physiological function, including the important process of fat metabolism, decreases. Dehydration can make your body go in search of water, signaling you to eat more, a phenomenon I call "artificial hunger." Dehydration also causes your digestive system to work at a diminished capacity, potentially preventing you from getting the nutrients you need and triggering unnecessary eating to make up for the shortfall. On the other hand, if you drink adequate amounts of water throughout the day, it'll not only keep all systems functioning smoothly, it'll fill you up, helping to curb your appetite so you eat relatively less, not more.

It's especially important to be hydrated when you exercise; your body can't cool itself adequately when it's low on fluid. What's more, being adequately hydrated during exercise will help you stay energized so that you can maintain an appropriate intensity and not quit early, and end up burning fewer calories both during and after your exercise session.

If you can work up to drinking nine eight-ounce glasses of water a day, great. But at the very least, try to get up to eight glasses—you'll need at least that much if you're moderately active. (When you exercise more and at a higher intensity, you may need even more.) Most people drink only when they're thirsty, but by the time you feel thirsty, your body may be already dehydrated. Drink water throughout the day, and don't consume too much at once: drinking more than one to two glasses at one sitting stimulates the body to rid itself of the water.

Your water requirement is over and above the water you get from foods such as soup and other beverages. What counts as water? Fresh, noncarbonated water. Carbonated (or sparkling) water, which can have somewhat of a diuretic effect, doesn't count. Neither do drinks that contain caffeine or alcohol, for the same reason. Remember, active people need more fluids than people who don't exercise, and pure water is your best source.

How to Work More Water into Your Day

- **Start the day with a glass of water.** Drink another glass before you work out, then two afterwards. Have another one a half hour before lunch, then one at lunch, and you'll already have had six glasses by midday.

- **Buy a water filter for your home.** Filtering makes your water taste better. It's also safer than drinking unfiltered water and cheaper than buying bottled water.

- **Carry a bottle of water with you at all times.** You don't have to buy bottled water to do this; just use a refillable sports bottle.

- **Any time you see a water fountain, stop and take a few sips.** Every little bit helps!

2. Working Out Aerobically

GOAL: Perform aerobic exercise for a minimum of 50 to 150 minutes per week, depending on your goals.

Aerobic exercise—the kind of exercise that makes your heart beat faster and your breathing accelerate—is one of the cornerstones of an effective weight loss program. For most people, changing their eating behavior means eating fewer calories, a move that can cause their metabolism to drop. If you bolster your metabolism with regular aerobic exercise and *then* begin to gradually eliminate unnecessary calories, your weight loss results will be dramatic.

That, though, is only one of several significant reasons for adding aerobic exercise to your life. Aerobic exercise improves cardiovascular fitness. That is, it improves the ability of your heart, lungs, and arteries to deliver oxygen to working muscles, as well as your muscles' ability to use that oxygen to fuel its efforts. By getting your cardiovascular system into shape, you'll bump up the total number of calories you burn in a day. You'll also receive the other perks of cardiovascular fitness: lower cholesterol, reduced risk of heart disease (and some cancers), better toned muscles, increased energy, and a more shapely body, just to name a few!

What Kind of Aerobic Exercise?

When weight loss is your goal, it's critical to choose a form of aerobic exercise that is *highly* aerobic. The more highly aerobic an activity is, the more aerobic enzymes it will cause your body to produce. These enzymes, found mostly in the muscles, help you burn fat, so you want your body to produce as many of them as possible.

The workouts that I consider the most effective forms of aerobic exercise—my A list—are powerwalking, jogging, aerobic dancing, and stair *climbing.* On the B list are stair *stepping,* elliptical exercise, spinning, stationary cycling, indoor rowing, and indoor cross-country skiing. Other workouts can help keep you healthy and contribute to weight loss, but these give you the most bang for your buck.

How Much?

One well-kept secret is that many of the beautiful bodies you see in movies, on TV, and in magazines, are the products of hours and hours of exercise. It's not that the glamorous owners of these bodies aren't busy, but often before being photographed they put a considerable amount of time into refining their shapes. It's part of their job.

In the real world, most people don't have that much time to devote to exercise, and I'm not expecting you to work out for hours at a time. But if your goal is to lose weight, you'll typically need to do *at least* fifty minutes a week of aerobic exercise. (Many people need to do more.) You can break up those minutes to best fit your schedule, but keep in mind that you'll need to do at least ten minutes of continuous exercise at a time to make any appreciable increase in your aerobic enzymes and thus your metabolism. If you hit a plateau in your weight loss, try adding more minutes of exercise each week; that should stimulate your body to start shedding pounds again.

How Hard?

The more aerobic work you perform in a given amount of time, the better cardiovascular shape you'll be in and the less body fat you'll retain. Perhaps you've heard that if you want to burn fat, you should stick to low-intensity exercise, but the rationale behind that recommendation is faulty. It's true that at higher intensities your body tends to burn more carbohydrates (in the form of glycogen, stored in the muscles and liver) than it does stored body fat. However, it doesn't matter that much *which* fuel you burn the most of during exercise. What does matter is that by exercising at a higher intensity you'll increase your metabolism, thus burning a higher rate of calories 24 hours a day!

The difference in the amount of fat you burn if you go slowly for thirty minutes and the amount you burn if you go at a moderately high pace for thirty minutes is pretty negligible. But the difference between the amount of fat your body will burn if you have a highly fit cardiovascular system and a system that's just so-so is significant. In the end, a revved-up metabolism will play a bigger part in ridding your body of excess fat than a low-intensity workout ever could.

So what is the ideal intensity? One that gets you "in the zone." Being in the zone means exercising at 70 to 80 percent of your maximum ability. There are two ways to figure out if you're reaching that goal.

The first method is a numerical equation that calculates what's known as your "target heart rate range." This is the recommended range of heartbeats per minute that you should achieve during exercise in order to train your cardiovascular system safely. To estimate your target heart rate range at 75 percent of your maximum ability, start by figuring out your target heart *rate:* 220 − your age × 75 percent (.75). So if you're forty years old, your target heart rate is 180 × .75 = 135 beats per minute. To get the target heart rate *range,* add and subtract 5 (beats) from your target heart rate. For a forty-year-old, that comes out to 130 to 140 beats per minute. So if you're forty, after you warm up for five minutes or so, your heart rate should be between 130 and 140 beats per minute for the duration of your workout.

The thing that's difficult about monitoring your heart rate this way is that you have to take your pulse during exercise, which can be sort of tricky. That's why I prefer that clients use the second method of determining if they're exercising in the zone: perceived exertion. (Of course, if you've been told by your physician not to exceed a certain heart rate, then stick with the first method.) Perceived exertion is a subjective measure of how hard you're working, based primarily on your breathing. The scale goes from zero to ten, with level zero being how it feels to be at rest and level ten being an exertion so difficult you could probably maintain it for only a few seconds. On this scale, being in the zone means being at level seven or eight. At level seven, you feel fatigue but are certain that you could maintain the pace for the rest of your session. Your breathing is deep, but you can still carry on a conversation. Level eight is slightly more vigorous. If you asked yourself if you could continue at that pace for the rest of your workout, you might not be 100 percent sure. You could still carry on a conversation, but you wouldn't feel like it.

It may take you a while to consistently maintain level seven, but don't be discouraged. If you can't exercise at that pace for your whole workout, start at a lower level of exertion, then increase to seven for one or two minutes at a time. Probably within a week or two you'll be able to exercise at level seven for at least ten to fifteen minutes. Remember that highly aerobic exercise isn't supposed to be completely comfortable. You need to challenge yourself if you want to see some results.

3. Eliminating Emotional Eating

GOAL: Begin to understand the causes of and eliminate your emotional eating.

No matter what you learn in this book about nutritious eating, it will be difficult for you to apply the information to your own life if you are struggling with emotional eating. If you sometimes (or often) eat because of how you *feel* rather than because you are truly *physically* hungry, you are an emotional eater. You may do it at meals, in between meals, at social occasions, or late at night (for more on the connection between emotional eating and late-night snacking, see page 42). You may do it for any number of reasons. Some people eat to comfort themselves in stressful situations. Some eat due to boredom and/or loneliness. Others eat when they experience turmoil or disappointment. Often people eat to fill a void when something or someone is missing from their lives.

Whenever you do it and whatever the reason, if you can eliminate emotional eating, you will achieve weight loss success and feel a greater sense of self-worth. Emotional eating is a viscious cycle. You eat to make yourself feel better but just end up making yourself feel worse by giving in to self-destructive impulses. But you *can* break the cycle. It *does* take time, and you must be gentle with yourself as you go along. However, with diligence, you can find other, healthier coping mechanisms and slowly but surely begin to understand and alter this behavior.

Overcoming emotional eating requires making some changes—some subtle, some bigger in scope. Here are the ones that I think will help you achieve success.

- **Organize your eating, and eat consciously.** When you don't have a plan, it's easier to give in to an emotional impulse and eat haphazardly. Limiting yourself to three meals and two snacks a day, as well as not eating at least two hours before bed, will give your day some structure. That structure will make it easier for you to take the time to enjoy each meal and snack as a conscious act. By a conscious act, I mean that you should make each meal an enjoyable event—whether it's with music and candles or just the company of someone you like. Reading, watching TV, or working while you eat doesn't allow you to register the experience and will leave you hungry and yearning for more food later on.

- **Learn the difference between physical hunger and emotional eating.** If you feed yourself out of emotional need, it's possible that you may have lost the ability to recognize what physical hunger feels like. Choose a day and delay your normally scheduled mealtime so that you can feel what it's like to be hungry. (If you have a medical condition such as diabetes, you must consult a physician before you try this.) Being familiar with this feeling will help you be a better judge of *why* you're eating whenever you eat. If you don't feel physical hunger, don't eat.

- **Identify the reasons why and occasions when you eat due to emotions.** If you're not hungry, why are you eating? This is an important question to ask yourself since it will help clue you in to what triggers your emotional eating episodes. I strongly suggest you keep a journal so that you can write down what you're feeling instead of eating. A journal is a great tool for identifying patterns and behaviors that you may not even be aware of—and of course you need to know what they are before you can change them! (See page 47 for more on keeping a journal.)

- **If you're depressed, consider seeking professional counseling.** There are many issues you may be able to deal with on your own and others that you can manage with the help of family and friends. But if you are continually and deeply depressed—or even if you just feel overwhelmed by life and need someone impartial to talk to—it's a good idea to seek the help of a professional counselor or therapist. For some people, this is a very hard step to take, but sometimes an outsider's insight is just what you need.

- **Use the moment of temptation to learn what needs to change in your life.** Eating can be an anesthetic. Sometimes people eat because they don't want to think, but thinking is *exactly* what I want you to do. Every time you're tempted to eat and you know it's not because you are physically hungry, you have a golden opportunity to learn something about yourself. Go to your journal. Think about why you are eating, and write it down. This is your chance for change—seize it!

- **Look for healthy outlets for your emotions.** There are many enriching alternatives to eating, and it may be helpful to keep a list of them handy to remind yourself of what they are. What do you like to do? It could be anything from reading a book to phoning a friend. Taking classes, taking up a craft, surfing the Web—all these can help. Perhaps the best substitute is exercise, even if it's only a walk around the block. Exercising won't just distract you, it will improve your mood and help counter the effects of stress.

4. Strength Training

GOAL: Incorporate strength training into your exercise routine three times a week.

Men and women have been strength training for years, but it's only recently that we've come to understand how beneficial strength training can be. If for no other reason, you should strength-train because it combats two profound effects of aging: muscle loss and bone loss. But strength training also has significant weight loss and weight maintenance benefits. The strength you gain from working with weights makes you capable of doing aerobic exercise at a higher level so that you ultimately burn more calories. Usually, lifting weights will also cause you to build muscle tissue, and since maintaining muscle requires a lot of energy, this will increase the number of calories you burn. At the very least, just by helping you retard age-related muscle loss, strength training will keep you from losing much of your body's natural calorie-burning ability.

When you strength-train, what you are essentially doing (or should be doing) is fatiguing your muscles to the point where they will rebuild themselves in order to handle the strain better next time around. Each exercise builds only certain muscles, so you need a regimen that includes exercises for all the major muscle groups in your body.

It's very important that no matter what strength training exercises you perform, you perform them properly. At the very least, bad form while exercising can cause aches and pains, and in the worst case it can cause injury. I give detailed instructions for an effective, easy-to-follow routine in *Get With the Program!*. You might also consider consulting a personal trainer or exercise specialist to teach you some weight lifting basics. If you do, I recommend that this person be certified by either the American College of Sports Medicine (ACSM), the American Council on Exercise (ACE), or the National Strength and Conditioning Association (NSCA).

How Often?

If you strength-train once a week, you will maintain your muscular strength, though your muscular endurance might decline some. Training two times a week will improve your muscular strength and more or less maintain your muscular endurance. Three times a week—the magic number—will improve both your muscular strength *and* your muscular endurance. (If you want to work up to four times a week, great, but it's not essential.)

How Many Sets and Repetitions?

A repetition (or rep) is one completion of a given exercise. If, for instance, you're doing a biceps curl, every time you raise the weight to your shoulder, then lower it back down to the starting position, you've completed one rep. Sets are groups of repetitions. I want you to do between eight and ten repetitions per set. Take a break between each set— but not too long a break. Limit your rest to fifteen to thirty seconds in-between sets. When you allow too much time to elapse, your muscles recover too quickly, lessening the effects of training. Begin by performing one set of each exercise; then, after about a month, progress to two sets. After another month, consider progressing to three sets.

How Much Weight?

To have an effect, the weights you use must cause fatigue in your muscles. But you don't want the weights to be so heavy that you strain yourself attempting to lift them. My suggestion is that you begin using a very light weight that you know you can lift without much effort. Increase this weight gradually until you arrive at a weight that makes you feel fatigued (or gives you a slight burning sensation in your muscles) after eight or ten repetitions. Before you go into your regular routine, do a warm-up set, which will help you avoid injury: using half the amount of weight that you've selected for the exercise, do four or five repetitions. Then proceed with the actual set.

Which Exercise?

The beauty of strength training is that it really doesn't take very much time and you don't have to do a million different exercises to get results. I've gotten great results with what I call the Essential Eight. These are basic exercises done with dumbbells that work all the major muscle groups and are relatively uncomplicated. If you're not familiar with strength training exercises, I refer you back to *Get With the Program!* or to an exercise professional for details. The Essential Eight are:

The Squat	The Butterfly
The Lunge	The Dumbbell Fly
The Chest Press	The Biceps Curl
The Shoulder Press	The Triceps Extension

PART II

The Guide to Good Eating

Four Steps to Good Eating

As you prepare to change the way you eat for a lifetime, I want to reiterate that you'll have the most success if you take each step one at a time and gradually weave them into your life. Attempting to adopt all four behaviors at the same time, while admirable, may well be self-defeating. If you take on more than you can reasonably handle, you may fail and lose your incentive to continue. It took you a long time to develop the behaviors you're trying to change, so go slow and wait for victory in each step before you tackle the next hurdle.

It's acceptable, even desirable, to take these four steps in the order that I've laid them out. I think that's the best (and the easiest) way to do it. But it's not absolutely necessary. You may find you want to start with Step 2 or 3. That's your choice. All I ask is that you not take on too much at one time. The best way to stay motivated is to meet one challenge, let your success inspire you, then take on the next one.

Step 1: Eat a Nutritious Breakfast

If you're thinking, "I'm not a breakfast eater, I can skip this section," you, more than anyone, need to keep on reading. Many people consider breakfast a kind of throwaway meal. They assume that skipping is a good way to cut calories and, since they're not really hungry in the morning anyway, a pretty painless way to lose weight at that. But the truth is that when you miss breakfast, you miss out on a great opportunity to boost your metabolism, raise your energy level, and positively influence the rest of your day's calorie intake. In fact, odd as it may sound, you're more likely to lose weight if you eat a couple of hundred calories in the morning than if you skip breakfast. Thus, far from being dispensable, breakfast is the most important meal of the day—*especially* if you're trying to lose weight.

How Eating Breakfast Revs You Up for the Day

A lot of work goes on inside you while you sleep; it's the time your body uses to repair and replenish itself. But one thing we're certain does not go on in full force is calorie burning. As far as we can tell, your metabolism starts slowing down at night so that you can fall asleep, slows even further as you slumber, then reaches its lowest point right before you wake up. By the time your eyes pop open at first light, you're hardly burning any calories at all. Your metabolism speeds up as the day wears on, but it's a gradual process—unless you make an effort to give it an immediate boost.

That's where breakfast comes in. Anytime you consume food, your body responds by raising the rate at which you burn calories. But when you eat breakfast, you get that boost early in the day, increasing the number of hours that your metabolism runs on high and, ultimately, the total number of calories you burn in a twenty-four-hour stretch. Exercising in the morning—whether you work out aerobically and/or strength-train—also raises your metabolism throughout the day. You'll get the biggest boost if you both eat breakfast and exercise in the morning: doing both increases the metabolism more than doing either one alone.

Another good reason to eat breakfast is that it elevates your energy level. Just as your metabolism is at a low ebb when you wake up in the morning, so is your blood sugar level. Blood sugar, also known as glucose, is what our bodies and brains use for energy; when it's low, you're likely to feel low energy, too, and as a consequence you won't do much.

And I don't just mean that you'll refrain from things like running up the stairs at the office or chasing the kids around the house. I mean that you'll end up economizing energy in simple ways that you're probably not even aware of. Maybe you'll sink into your chair rather than lean forward when you talk to someone. Perhaps you'll sit down rather than stand as you speak on the phone. These may seem like negligible energy expenditures, but the hundreds, even thousands, of little moves you make all day add up.

In fact, those small moves probably account for some of the difference between people who struggle with their weight and those who don't. When you put a camera in a room with people who are overweight and people who have been thin most or all of their lives, you can see that the thin people are dramatically more active. Everyone knows people who are kinetic, always buzzing around. All that buzzing means they're burning calories.

Breakfast is a great energizer that will help you approach both physical and mental tasks with increased vigor. Leave the house with something in your stomach, and you'll be better able to concentrate and solve problems. You'll feel less tired, and if you've always been sort of a morning grump, you'll probably be less irritable, too.

Earlier I said that eating breakfast would also have a positive influence on the rest of your day's calorie intake. That's because if you eat a meal—even a small one—first thing in the morning, it will help you stave off the impulse to overeat later in the day. Think about it. Assuming you have your night eating under control, you have your last bite of food around 8 P.M. You wake up at say, 7 A.M., go about your morning and late-morning routine, then sit down to lunch around noon. That's sixteen hours without food! Who *wouldn't* be ravenous? When you're that hungry, you set yourself up for an oversized lunch or dinner (or both!). However, had you taken the time to eat breakfast, you'd be on a more even keel and less likely to overeat. If you're a late-night eater, you may even find that eating breakfast dampens your after-hours cravings.

What If You're Not Hungry in the Morning?

When I bring up the topic of breakfast, some people are all ears—they could live on cereal, toast, and other typical breakfast foods. Most people, though, would rather not hear another word about it. "The morning is the one time I'm not hungry, and now you're asking me to eat? It seems to go against common sense."

I'm not sure why some of us wake up hungry, and some of us don't, but it could be that not waking up hungry is a sign of a slow metabolism. As I mentioned before, everyone's metabolism slows down significantly at night. In the morning, as you wake up, its rate increases, but if you have a naturally slow metabolism, it will increase at a snail's pace. So if you find you're not hungry until lunchtime, your metabolism is most likely to blame. Or else you ate too much the night before. That's actually the most common reason people don't feel hungry when they wake up in the morning. We'll deal with *that* problem when we get to Step 2.

Also, consider that your inclination to skip breakfast may just be sheer habit. If sitting down at the breakfast table was never stressed in your household when you were growing up, you're probably used to skipping it. Or maybe, as an adult, you've just felt too rushed in the morning to bother with breakfast and by now your body doesn't mind giving it a pass. In a sense, you've *trained* yourself not to be hungry. You may also just feel reluctant to break the habit because you think skipping breakfast is a good way to reduce your calorie intake. But again, that's a serious misconception; you'll probably wind up eating fewer total calories if you do eat breakfast.

FEAR OF BREAKFAST: EMILY'S STORY

Emily had been struggling with her weight since she was a teenager, but by the time she reached her mid-twenties she thought she'd found the perfect way to keep it under control. Her strategy was to have a cappuccino (with skim milk, of course) in the morning, perhaps a cup of yogurt for lunch, then eat a big dinner. Her dinner choices were generally healthy, but she ate way too much food. Not only that, but this schedule made her feel terrible. She was dragging all afternoon, and she felt out of control at dinnertime. The foods she chose to eat at night might have been nutritious, but she was so hungry that she ate portions that were ridiculously oversized.

When she finally sought help, Emily was advised that she would have to start eating breakfast, an idea that was literally painful to her. "Going from something to nothing was a huge leap," she remembers. But she started out slow. One day she'd have some dry toast and skim milk, the next a bowl of cereal. She waited to see if she'd gain weight, but to her surprise she didn't put on a pound. She did, though, feel much better. Ultimately, she readjusted her meals so that she wasn't eating such a heavy dinner, and even though she was taking in more calories, she stayed thin.

It's been about fifteen years since she first began eating in the morning, and she has had three children in the interim. She has maintained her weight and still eats breakfast, though she admits that eating in the morning is still sometimes hard. "But anytime I think about skipping breakfast now, I just remind myself that it will cause my metabolism to drop, and that keeps me eating."

Getting into the Breakfast Habit

If you're not used to eating first thing in the morning, you may have to cajole yourself to eat for three to six weeks before you begin feeling hungry and want to eat when you wake up. You may, however, need to ease into the habit. There's probably something you can visualize yourself eating in the morning. Start there. It might be as simple as a glass of juice, an apple or a slice of watermelon, or a single slice of toast with fruit spread. It doesn't even have to be what I consider a perfect breakfast and can be something you don't usually think of as a breakfast food, such as a handful of trail mix or some crackers and a slice of cheese. Think of it as a first step. Once you get accustomed to eating some kind of breakfast, you can explore healthier options.

Thwarting the Morning Time Crunch

A lot of people skip breakfast purely because of time constraints. Or at least they tell themselves they don't have time. Although I know that getting out of the house in the morning can be taxing, especially if you have kids, it's really not a good excuse for skipping breakfast. And it's an even worse excuse for eating junky "convenience" foods such as fat-laden muffins and donuts. Remember, children usually follow their parents' lead when it comes to eating. By sitting down to a nutritious breakfast yourself, you'll be setting a good example that will help them develop healthy habits and avoid weight problems of their own. Perhaps you're following the not-particularly-good example your parents set right now. Don't pass it on to another generation.

A healthful breakfast can be made in a matter of minutes. In only a few more seconds than it takes to unwrap a Danish, you can pour yourself a bowl of cereal with low-fat or skim milk or even scramble an egg. Allow yourself a few more minutes, and you can toast some whole-grain bread, slice up some cantaloupe, or blend yourself a fresh fruit smoothie (see page 106). But let's be honest. You already know that there are many healthful quick fixes you can make in the morning. Still, if for whatever reason you find that you're allowing time constraints to prevent you from eating a nutritious breakfast, you may need to re-think your priorities as well as your daily routine.

Help Yourself Become a Breakfast Eater

- **Renew your commitment to yourself every morning.** The beginning of each day is a perfect time to remind yourself to get with the program. Eating breakfast is the first step in the plan that you've promised yourself you'd stick with.

- **Get up fifteen minutes earlier.** Fifteen minutes is really a drop in the bucket in terms of sleep, but it's more than enough time to squeeze breakfast into your morning ritual. If, psychologically, it will help you get up earlier, go to bed fifteen minutes earlier.

- **Organize your day as you eat.** In general, I believe that it's better to keep your mind on the experience of eating when you're having a meal. If you watch TV or read while you eat, you'll end up just throwing food down and losing track of how much you're consuming, and, because you're not really registering or enjoying the experience, you may feel deprived later. But I make an exception for breakfast, particularly for people who usually skip the meal because they feel as though their time is better spent doing other things to prepare for their day. If that's your M.O., I suggest that, as you eat, you organize your day, writing down what you need to accomplish. By giving yourself those few minutes to itemize what you need to do, breakfast can help you save, not waste, time.

The Best Breakfast

In terms of the nutrient makeup of a meal—that is, how much carbohydrate, protein, and fat it contains—I don't believe that there really is such a thing as a perfect meal, because each meal has to figure into the context of what you eat during the rest of the day. So, in a sense, it doesn't matter if your breakfast is high in carbohydrates and low in protein and fat because you still have an opportunity to get the protein and fat you need later in the day.

Actually, active people can get away with eating a higher percentage of carbohydrates in the morning partially because carbs are a primary fuel for exercise. If you work out before breakfast, you'll need to replace the glycogen that you've just used. But even if you didn't exercise pre-

The Case for Working Out in the Morning

When you exercise is less important than *if* you exercise. Just doing it is the most important thing of all. That said, however, there are a couple of reasons I'm an advocate of morning workouts. The first has to do with metabolism. Whether you go for a power walk at 7 A.M. or 7 P.M., you will still burn approximately the same amount of calories during the workout (provided, of course, that you do it for the same distance and at the same pace). You will also raise your metabolic rate for some time after both workouts—but in the morning you will boost it higher, netting you more calories burned over the course of a day.

What accounts for the difference? When you exercise in the morning, you have a full day to operate with your metabolism revved up. However, at night, your metabolism is in the process of slowing down as part of your body's preparation for sleep. Even though exercise adds some stimulus, it's not enough to override the reduction of your body's calorie-burning rate. As a consequence, you never get that extended accelerated burnoff.

Another reason that I'm a proponent of morning exercise is that getting a workout under your belt early will give you a sense of accomplishment and help inspire you to stay committed to the program for the remainder of the day. Research also shows that people who work out in the morning are more likely to be regular exercisers than are people who exercise at night. If you think about it, it makes a lot of sense. If you plan your workouts for the morning, there's usually less to get in your way. But if you plan to exercise in the evening, a million things can pop up to let you off the hook—including the fact that by day's end you just feel too wiped out to work out. It's not absolutely necessary to exercise in the morning; you have to choose a time that's appropriate for your individual schedule and capabilities. However, if you have the opportunity, I definitely recommend giving it a try.

breakfast, carbohydrates will charge you up more quickly than protein and fat. Think of them as the good fuel for starting your engine in the morning.

The size of your breakfast is another factor to consider. Most people don't eat very much in the morning, so overeating generally isn't a problem, but you should be aware that overly large meals can make your body store fat. When you eat a large number of calories at one sitting, your body secretes an abnormally high amount of insulin. This is commonly referred to as an insulin spike. Insulin's job is to take blood glucose out of the bloodstream and lay it down as body fat—exactly what you *don't* want to happen.

To avoid an insulin spike, it's best to consume 25 to 30 percent of your total daily calories at each meal, with the remaining 10 to 25 percent coming from snacks. You don't have to get out a pencil or a calculator, but try to shoot for something close to that division. In an ideal world, all of our meals would be equal, containing about a third of a day's calories, but few people want to eat that big a breakfast. I'll talk more about redistributing your calories throughout the day in a later section.

As to the quality of your breakfast, avoid saturated and trans-fats and foods that have been processed with so many additives and preservatives that their ingredient listings read like a chemist's manual. Choose whole-grain breads and cereals over those made with refined grains, and be aware of the sugar content of the foods you eat. Breakfast cereals in particular—even those that aren't noticeably frosted—can be jam-packed with sugar and unnecessary calories. You'll be better off choosing a no-sugar or low-sugar cereal and sweetening it with fruit (see page 108 for a great granola recipe). If you must sprinkle a teaspoon of sugar on top, you'll still end up using less than if you purchased a presweetened cereal. Fruit, though, has plenty of natural sugar and if you buy good-quality, in-season fruit, you'll find that you can really taste its sweetness. Eventually you'll find that you crave the sweetness of fruit and that the taste of a presweetened cereal will be too sugary. The same thing goes for yogurt. Get used to enhancing plain yogurt with fruit instead of buying the kind with fruit (and sugar) already added.

Coffee (or tea) is a morning ritual I won't ask you to give up, although I will say that it's in your best health interest to keep your caffeine intake to a minimum. I'm a coffee drinker myself, though I've been gradually phasing it out of my life. I used to drink too much throughout the day, but three years ago I cut back, and recently, I've cut back even further so that now I drink only one cup of coffee in the morning. Anytime I want something hot after that, I drink chamomile tea. I feel better and sleep better, too. Try to limit your own intake to one or two cups of caffinated coffee or tea in the morning, then switch to herbal teas later in the day.

Quick-and-Easy Breakfast Options

The breakfast recipes you'll find beginning on page 105 are not difficult or terribly time-consuming. They're delicious and healthy, and I hope you will try all of them. However, I realize that on some days you may need something quicker to get you out of the house, so here are a few ideas for fast fixes. They require just minutes to prepare, and some can even be eaten on the run—so no more protests that you don't have time for breakfast!

Fruit salad sprinkled with chopped walnuts or almonds
Seven-grain toast with fruit spread
A handful of trail mix
Frozen whole-grain toaster waffles with fruit spread
Instant oatmeal or other whole-grain hot cereal with sliced bananas and blueberries
Half an English muffin with melted low-fat cheese
A soft-boiled egg on a piece of whole-wheat toast

A hard-boiled egg

An egg-white sandwich

A peanut butter sandwich

Low-fat or fat-free yogurt with berries

Whole-grain cereal with skim milk (try to choose a cereal with no added sugar)

Apple or pear slices topped with low-fat cheese

A quesadilla—a corn tortilla topped with melted low-fat cheese

Eating and Exercise

Should you eat before you exercise in the morning or after? This is a very individual matter. I myself definitely need a little something before I work out, so I'll have a half slice of whole-wheat toast with fruit spread, a little bit of fresh fruit, or even a small shot of grapefruit juice. Then, when I'm done exercising, I'll go back and have a full breakfast.

I'm aware, though, that this might not work for everybody, especially those of you who already have trouble forcing something down in the morning. So while I think it's a good idea to give your body some fuel before exercising, you'll have to see what works for you. As you become fitter, I think you'll find that you do need something to get you through your workout. After exercise, you can eat a breakfast that includes a good amount of carbohydrates: your metabolism will be in high gear and will burn them easily.

If your schedule is flexible enough, you might even consider eating a full breakfast, waiting a bit, then exercising. How long should you wait? It depends. Some people need to wait longer than others, and if you work out too soon after eating, you may get a stitch in your side. Say, for instance, you go running ten minutes after a meal. Both your digestive system and your muscles need oxygen to do their jobs and they'll engage in a tug of war to get the most O_2. And guess what's going to win? Your legs. That will make it difficult to digest the food you just ate and leave you vulnerable to a stitch.

A good rule of thumb is to wait at least thirty minutes after eating to exercise. You may find you're able to handle exercising even sooner after you've eaten. But everybody is different, so experiment a little to see how long you need to wait.

Step 2: Set an Eating Cutoff Time

When I was a kid, I loved daylight saving time because it stayed light long enough for me to go out to play after dinner. I wasn't aware of it back then, but I'm certain that I burned off almost everything I'd just eaten. Adults, of course, don't usually go out to play after dinner, even during daylight saving time, and they often don't eat as early as kids do. Many adults, in fact, have a late dinner and turn in a short time afterward or else snack close to bedtime. Either way, they take in calories at a time when they're least likely to burn them off.

To succeed at weight loss, you'll need to stop eating two, preferably three, hours before going to sleep. You may feel slightly hungry, but that's exactly how I want you to feel. I never want you to feel ravenous when you go to bed at night. But wanting a little something is just fine. When you're trying to lose weight, slipping into bed at night feeling slightly hungry (the British have a perfect word for it—peckish) is actually a good thing. It's your body telling you that what you did that day is working—you're losing body fat. If you don't feel this way, you're probably not losing fat.

Start with a cutoff time of two hours before bed; then, as it becomes easier, see if you can stop eating two and a half hours presleep. If you can make it to three hours, even better. This little step can have a big payoff. A large percentage of my clients have found that establishing a cutoff time was all they needed to do to meet their weight loss goals. Others have needed to make additional changes as well, but everybody who quit late-night eating found that it translated into some weight loss. If you want to shed some pounds, go to bed feeling a little peckish. I'm confident that you'll see results.

Why It's Good to Be Just a Little Hungry at Bedtime

I want to reiterate that I don't advocate going to bed feeling starved. If you are voraciously hungry, it means that you didn't do a good job of managing your meals throughout the day. Perhaps you skipped breakfast or another meal, or maybe you just skimped on calories all day long. Either way, you may feel virtuous, but it just means that you missed a number of opportunities to give your metabolism a boost by eating. It also means that by allowing yourself to get ravenous, you may be setting yourself up for a binge. What I want you to feel instead is *slight* hunger. That feeling is your brain saying, "Feed me or I'm going to dip into your fat stores for energy." That, of course, is exactly what you want to happen. It's your guarantee that your body is burning the fat you are working hard to lose.

If, on the other hand, you follow your brain's directive and eat close to bedtime, your body will not dip into the fat it has stored away, and will probably even store some more. As I mentioned before, every time you eat, your metabolism increases slightly. But this effect is lost or minimized late at night. You don't get the same metabolism-boosting benefit when you eat just before bed, because a couple of hours after dinner, your body begins preparing for sleep. This natural slackening of your metabolic rate overrides any metabolic boost you might get from eating. So once you hit the pillow, the only calories you're going to use are the basic calories you need to keep your heart beating and your lungs breathing and allow your eyes to move in REM sleep. And that, all told, is a minimal number of calories.

You also won't take advantage of the energizing effects of eating. Had you eaten 300 calories in the morning instead of just before going to sleep, you'd feel invigorated and would move more throughout the day, burning those calories. But when you're downshifting into bed-time mode, you're going to feel too sleepy to increase your activity. The opportunity to burn off those 300 calories is lost.

Believe it or not, eating late at night can also inhibit your calorie-burning potential the next day. Say, for instance, that you treat yourself to a big bowl of cereal topped with sliced bananas at 10 P.M. one night and are fast asleep by eleven. When your alarm goes off the next morn-ing at seven, the last thing on your mind is going to be breakfast—you're still full from the cereal and bananas you ate the night before. Chances are, you're going to skip breakfast and lose all the metabolism-boosting benefits you'd get from eating a morning meal.

During sleep, digestion all but shuts down so that the food you've consumed has extended contact time with your digestive tract. That may increase your risk of various ailments and disease, including cer-tain cancers. Consider, too, that fat and protein takes longer than car-bohydrate to digest so if you snack on a bowl of ice cream or a steak sandwich before bed, the contact time may be even longer. Eating late can also just make you feel plain lousy. It's harder to get a good night's sleep on a full stomach, and it makes you more susceptible to heart-burn.

TWO TYPES OF LATE-NIGHT EATERS

JENNY'S STORY: Like a lot of people with time-consuming jobs, Jenny would get home from work well into the evening, sometimes not until 9 P.M. She'd then proceed to have dinner and, while her meals weren't catastrophically caloric—sometimes she'd have soup and bread, other times a few crab cakes—they still contained an ample number of calories. But that wasn't the problem. The problem was that because she had to get up early to go back to work the next day, she'd go to bed shortly after dinner.

When I began working with Jenny, I asked her to adopt an eat-ing cutoff time, and she was very open to the idea. The first thing she did was redesign her dinner schedule. Instead of eating a meal when she got home on the evenings that she worked late, Jenny made a point of having dinner while still at the office (fortunately, she worked in a place where she was able to have healthful food delivered.) At my suggestion, she also stopped what she was doing when the food came, cleared off her desk, and allowed herself to enjoy the meal—a critical step in helping her feel satisfied and less likely to go rooting through her cupboards when she got home later.

The second and ultimately more important thing that Jenny did was to start questioning her work life. Why was she at the office so late every night? Looking at her eating habits made her look at her work habits, and she realized she was working her life away. She cut back on her hours at the office by cutting out unnecessary meetings from her schedule. That helped her have dinner at a more reasonable time and to spend more time with her friends and boyfriend. Combined with eating in-office meals on the occasional nights when she still had to work late, that did the trick: Jenny quickly lost ten pounds.

SUZANNE'S STORY: When Suzanne first came to me hoping to lose the fifteen extra pounds she'd been carrying around, I had trouble figuring out why she was overweight. She was a dedicated exerciser and maintained a nearly perfect diet. But then I found out that two or three times a week, she would binge right before bedtime. And I mean *really* binge. Suzanne was capable of downing a pint of premium ice cream (the kind that's super high in fat) or half a bakery cake at one sitting. Because she ate a normal number of calories throughout the day, it was clear to me that these eating episodes were related not to physical hunger, but rather to emotional hunger. And as I got to know her better, I discovered that she indeed had a void in her life.

The nighttime binges had begun after she got divorced and

had continued through several years of unsatisfying dates and relationships. To stop the binges, Suzanne needed to first make the connection between her eating and her love life, then find a way to get fulfillment from something other than food. It took a lot of hard work. She started keeping a journal to help her understand the feelings that triggered binges and seeing a therapist to talk about the void in her life. A year later, she met a man and got remarried. By this time she had stopped her bingeing and, not surprisingly, had lost the extra fifteen pounds.

Habitual and Emotional Eating

Occasionally, I come across someone who snacks late at night out of true physical hunger—someone, that is, who just doesn't organize her meals well and as a result really feels the need to eat late into the evening. But mostly I see late-night snackers who eat out of habit and snackers who are emotional eaters, who eat to anesthetize themselves.

I used to fall into the habitual snacker category. I often tell the story of how, when I was growing up, my family would sit down together before bed and have a communal prebedtime snack. My mom, dad, sister, and I, usually clad in our pajamas, would gather around the table and have something like milk and cookies, ice cream, or hot chocolate, then roll off to bed happy and full. Back then, it seemed like a healthy thing to do, especially if the snack involved milk, which we were told would help us sleep (that part, at least, is somewhat true, since milk contains the natural sedative tryptophan). But to me, the best nights involved pie. I loved it then, and I love it now! To this day, whenever I'm offered a slice, I'm tempted to indulge and have a hard time passing it up. But I suspect that's mostly because I associate it with those intimate, comforting evenings I spent with my family.

I still crave that comforting ritual, but I've found a fulfilling substitute for the sweets: chamomile tea. I really relish that time of day when I'm able to sit down with something warm and calming, and the tea-drinking ritual allows me to preserve my family tradition—though in a much healthier (and far less caloric) way. When I go to bed, I feel satisfied but not stuffed the way I used to. As a result, I fall asleep more easily and get a better night's sleep.

Habit was half of my problem; emotional attachment to the tradition was the other half. I find that many people share this emotional attachment to late-night eating. They're not physically hungry when they eat; they're using food for emotional sustenance. Many of these emotional eaters do okay during the day, but at night they have time to reflect on what's wrong in their lives, and that sets the ball rolling. Suddenly, stress, anger, sadness—all the things that have been hidden under the surface during the day—boil over, leaving them desperate for something to wash the discomfort away. Food, handy and comforting, seems like the perfect remedy, but it's really just a bandage that masks, not solves, the problem. In fact, most emotional eaters ultimately find little pleasure in their late-night snacks, and they feel worse knowing that they're adding to their weight problems with every bite.

There are various degrees of emotional eating. Some people just feel a little discontented (or bored), so they'll eat a few cookies to distract themselves for a while. Others are in deep pain, which leads them to seriously abuse food. For them, it takes a lot more than cookies to fill the void they feel inside.

But whichever category you fall into—or perhaps you fall somewhere in between—it's imperative to address the reasons behind your emotional eating. In order to lose weight, you have to have a healthy relationship with food, and that means seeing food for what it is—a source of sustenance, nutrition, and enjoyment, but *not* a source of emotional fulfillment.

I don't want this to sound flippant, as if I think it's easy to give up using food for solace. I know it's not, and I don't want you—and this is important—to feel guilty or distressed about your desire to eat. But I *do* want to encourage you to seize this chance to understand *why* you turn to food. It's an incredible opportunity to change your life significantly. Working on your weight is actually working on your life—and that's what *Get With the Program!* is all about. Get in touch with your inner self, and the outer self will follow.

Dealing with the Discomfort of Being a Little Hungry

If your day goes according to plan, you'll expend more energy than you consume. And that's great—it means that you will burn body fat. It also means that, at least in the beginning, you will feel a twinge of hunger at night. If you're not used to it, it can make you very uncomfortable. This is a time when you really need to hang in there. As you become used to adhering to an eating cutoff time, your body will adapt and the uncomfortable feelings will pass.

It's just like training your body through exercise: the first day that you laced up your sneakers, put the treadmill on a hill setting, and began walking, you probably felt uncomfortable (and probably didn't like it). But that's what exercise training is: the gradual introduction of slight discomfort in order to make changes such as enhanced cardiovascular efficiency, greater muscle strength, and a stronger body overall. Another of those changes is increased tolerance. After jumping on the treadmill many times, it's going to feel less taxing; your body has adapted to the positive stress. You'll think back to the time when you were walking on a flat treadmill at a much pokier speed and wonder how you could have ever thought it was hard!

There are many other areas of our lives where we start out feeling uncomfortable with something, only, over time, to get to a point where it doesn't bother us—we may even come to like it. I remember once going out to dinner with a client who raved about the restaurant's asparagus soup. It was very rich and creamy, but since this was her last hurrah before we started to work together, she decided to order it. And she wasn't disappointed. To her, it tasted great.

Fast-forward to a year later. By this time we had weaned her from a diet of mostly rich, high-fat foods, but when we went back to the

How a Journal Can Help

I'm a big fan of initially keeping track of your food intake, your daily activities, and your thoughts and feelings throughout the day. For the first two to three months of a weight loss program, keeping a journal benefits just about everyone. It is especially helpful if you're an emotional eater, giving you insight into what's going on in your head when your stomach tells you to eat. I go into the details of keeping a journal in both *Get With the Program!* and *Get With the Program! Daily Journal,* but here are some basics that might help you get started.

- Keep your journal where it's easily accessible, and write down how you're feeling whenever you get the urge to eat. (If you can't carry it with you, keep it on your nightstand so that even if you don't record your day hour by hour, you can write a recap before turning in at night.)

- It may take a while, but over time you'll probably see a pattern emerge that will help you better understand why you're tempted to eat and help you differentiate between real physical hunger and the false tug of emotional hunger. Maybe your mind is reeling from a bad day at the office. Maybe your body is reeling because you skipped a meal or two. With practice, you'll learn which is which, and knowing will help make it easier for you to exercise control. Next time, before automatically reaching for the cookie jar, you'll be able to ask yourself, "Physical or emotional hunger?" and get a straight answer. This might not always keep you from eating out of emotional hunger, but it's a beginning that will likely lead to change.

- Looking at your life and asking yourself, "What do I need to change?" is one of the hardest things you'll ever have to do. But if you have the courage to take a clear-eyed look at your life, the rewards will be great. Even if you can't alter everything overnight—and you shouldn't expect to—you can get on the road to change. Just being on that road will help you feel better about yourself and make it easier to keep going. Each step you take will motivate you to take the next one and the next one after that, until, eventually, you reach your goals.

restaurant, she decided to order the asparagus soup again. Only this time she found it totally unappetizing. Her palate had become much more sensitized to fat, so that what used to taste delicious now tasted too rich.

It works this way with a lot of foods. Switch from heavily salted dishes to lightly salted dishes, and after a while, you'll probably find the heavily salted versions too hard to take. You'll be so sensitive to sodium that you'll even start tasting the natural sodium contained in foods such as broccoli. It works the opposite way, too. Keep adding salt to your food, and you'll eventually become desensitized to it—you won't taste the salt even though it's there in abundance.

There's a word for the process of going through a period of discomfort, then adjusting to what's causing the stress; habituation. When continually exposed to just about anything we have the ability to adjust and develop a tolerance. That's what going to happen when you begin nixing late-night eating. You'll find it uncomfortable at first, but you'll adjust. Yet even though your body has this remarkable ability to adapt, I still suggest that you take it slowly. Start with a two-hour cutoff time and honor it. Then see how much further you can cut back. Go to two and a half hours. If you can make it to three, great! Have patience, and you will prevail.

Tips for Thwarting Late-Night Snacking

- **Replace a late-night snack with a cup of herbal tea.** This, as you know, is my personal strategy, but I find that it also works for a lot of other people. The warmth of a cup of herbal tea (I find chamomile especially calming) is comforting, and the liquid helps give you a feeling of fullness. And if it's boredom that is driving you to eat, the tea will help keep you busy until the urge to eat passes. The ritual of tea drinking also gives you time to reflect on your day and set your personal goals for tomorrow.

- **Write!** You might even combine writing with tea drinking, since tea can put you in a contemplative mood. But even if you're not a tea drinker, writing is a good way to foil late-night snacking. Jot down what you're feeling—it may convince you that maybe what you need is not a bag of potato chips but a phone call to a good friend to talk about what's bothering you. Write about the ways you want to improve your life and what you think can help you do so.

- **Keep yourself busy.** Boredom is the enemy of all late-night eaters. Read a book, watch a movie (though not if you're the kind of person who associates TV with snacking), take a bath, challenge someone in your family to a card game, listen to music, put pictures in a photo album, surf the Internet. If it's safe, go for a walk by yourself or with someone else. Choose something that enriches your life in some way so that it's not simply a substitute for eating that you will ultimately throw aside. If the activity you opt for is absorbing and enriching, your cravings will most likely dissipate.

- **Close the day by renewing your commitment to yourself.** You did it first thing in the morning; now do it again at night. Review your day. What did you do right? What needs to change?

Step 3: Redistribute Your Calories

When you're trying to lose weight, how much you eat matters. Everyone knows that. But *when* you eat also matters, though that's a piece of the weight loss puzzle that's often overlooked. The eating schedule most people maintain today goes something like this: they skip breakfast, have a small lunch, then do their power eating at dinner. It may not sound so bad on the surface, but in fact it's a perfect prescription for putting on pounds.

On the other hand, a day that looks more like this—a healthy-size meal for breakfast, a moderate lunch, one or two snacks during the day, and a small dinner—is the perfect prescription for taking off pounds. Exactly how many pounds you'll drop by redistributing your calories this way will depend on your individual body (and how you were patterning your meals before), but you will lose weight. One example of how well it works is a client of mine who shed eight stubborn pounds in nine weeks simply by reproportioning the size of her meals. She didn't eat less food than before; she just ate more of it earlier in the day.

I've already talked a little bit about how eating raises your metabolism and energy level, and how consuming a large number of calories at once can increase your body's propensity to store fat. But let's recap here so that you can see what these physiological effects have to do with redistributing your calories.

Four Physiological Reasons to Spread Out Your Calories

1   **The more frequently you eat, the more often you'll give your metabolism a boost.** You might think that you're doing yourself a favor by skipping meals. You might even feel as though you're doing yourself a favor by not eating until dinner. But physiology dictates that eating—and eating often—is actually a better strategy. Eating has a stimulating effect on the metabolism, increasing the rate at which you burn calories for some time after a meal. Eat often, and your metabolism will operate at its maximum speed all day long.

2   **Calories eaten earlier in the day boost the metabolism more than calories eaten later in the day.** When you eat, you increase the rate at which you burn calories, but your metabolism still has a natural arc to it and it declines as it gets closer to bedtime. For that reason, it may be that the food you eat in the evening doesn't increase your calorie-burning ability as much as the food you eat earlier in the day. Once it's settled into its resting mode, your body is resistant to being revved up at night.

3 **Eating makes you feel more energetic during the day but not, typically, at night.** Have you ever finished dinner and thought to yourself, "I feel as if I could run a few miles!" I didn't think so. Most people feel fairly lethargic after dinner. One reason is that they've usually eaten too much and their bodies are hard at work digesting the food, leaving little energy for anything else. (This is especially true when the meal is high in fat and protein, which take more energy to digest than carbohydrates.) Another is that the body begins to wind down in the evening, preparing you for sleep.

4 **Eating the majority of your calories at one meal can create an insulin spike, causing the body to store fat.** When you take in a large number of calories—and, in particular, carbohydrate calories—a signal is sent to your brain, which then sends a message to your pancreas to pump out more insulin. That big dose of insulin is going to cause your body to store many of those calories as fat (insulin, you'll remember, is responsible for taking glucose out of the bloodstream and depositing it into fat storage). The majority of people eat their biggest meal at dinner time, but having an oversized meal any time of day can cause an insulin spike. If, however, you spread out the calories over many hours, your insulin level will stay steady and your body will be less likely to hoard fat.

Downsizing Dinner

Don't be surprised if you find that one of the hardest parts of redistributing your calories is downsizing dinner. Some things are sacred in American life, and dinner is definitely one of them. Dinner is the meal that we put the most thought into, and from a gastronomic standpoint, dinner dishes are the foods we take most seriously. (How often do restaurant critics review an eatery's lunch or breakfast offerings? Almost never.) Perhaps even more important, dinner is the time when we sit down with family or friends to socialize and discuss how the day went. After a long day of working or caring for the home, it's a great reward.

Yet dinner is also key in determining how much you weigh. Sitting down to a big meal at night is the equivalent of putting a big cash deposit into a bank right before it closes: it'll be too late for the bank to pay out any checks, so the cash will just be tucked away in the vault. If, on the other hand, you make a big deposit in the morning, the bank has the entire day to pay out checks. Likewise, if you consume most of your calories in the early part of the day, your body will have time to burn them. But if you consume the bulk of your calories at dinner, you'll have no opportunity to expend them. Like the end-of-the-day cash deposit, they'll get tucked away in the vault—your fat cells.

Remember, too, that if you blow it by overeating earlier in the day, you still have several hours to work it off. And I don't mean you'll have to get back on the StairMaster because you had too much to eat at lunch. Rather, since eating has elevated your energy level, you'll probably just naturally burn it off. You'll get up to pick up a book instead of just reaching for it, sit more erectly, walk faster—unconsciously move differently in hundreds of little ways that will have a big calorie-burning impact.

But if you overeat at dinner, you can't make up for it. It's a done deal. As I mentioned when I talked about having an eating cutoff time at night, it's better to feel as though you could still eat a little something before sleep than to go bed on a full stomach. Look for that feeling; it's your assurance that you're at a calorie deficit. This has become something of a mantra, I know, but it bears repeating: that slight tug of hunger is your body warning you that if you don't feed it, it's going to dip into your fat stores—exactly what you want to happen!

None of this is to say that dinner shouldn't still play an important role in your life. However, your evening meal doesn't have to be enormous to have significance. This is a time when it's really important to practice portion control. Dine on foods that you love and make the eating experience worthwhile, but consume these foods in moderation.

And focus on the social aspect of the meal rather than making the food the most important part of your day. Think of the ritual of dinner not just as a source of physical sustenance but emotional sustenance as well, a time to connect with the people with whom you're sharing the meal. And if you're dining alone? Still take the time to make it special. Light candles, put on music, make it an enjoyable event.

Why Snacking Is a Good Thing

In the days before we knew much about metabolism and some of the other weight loss facts we know now, snacking was taboo. If you snacked, it was thought, you lacked willpower and were probably not going to lose the weight you were trying to. But now we realize that, when it's not produced by *emotional* hunger, the desire to snack can be a sign that your metabolism is humming along, burning calories as it should. Of course, your success depends on what you snack on—if you treat yourself to a box of donuts and then some a few times a day, no, you probably won't lose weight.

Snacks can serve a couple of purposes. Just like meals, they give your metabolism a little boost so that you burn more calories. Snacks also give you an energy lift. If you don't eat anything when you start feeling sluggish at three in the afternoon, you'll sit in your chair all foggy-headed, doing nothing. But if you have a reasonable snack—reasonable meaning about 75 to 150 calories and preferably containing both protein and carbohydrate—you'll charge up and probably snap out of it in about ten or fifteen minutes.

Another benefit of snacking is that it will help you spread out your calories so that you don't overeat at any one meal. It may even help to think of your snacks as part of the preceding meal, just eaten later. You might, for instance, save the toast you were going to have with your cereal during breakfast and eat it at midmorning instead. Or hold on to the yogurt you were going to eat right after lunch, and make it your 3 P.M. snack.

Be aware, though, that sometimes our bodies fool us with what I

What Do Well-Distributed Calories Look Like?

You should eat three meals—breakfast, lunch, and dinner—plus two snacks—midmorning and midafternoon—a day. I suggest that you try to make each meal 25 to 30 percent of your total daily calories, with snacks making up the remaining 10 to 25 percent. The size of the portions will vary according to the number of calories you individually need to eat in a day. If you're inclined to make one meal bigger than the others, make that larger meal lunch. That way you'll still have half a day to burn off the extra calories.

The recipes in the back of this book can be combined to create a well-proportioned day of eating. Just below, though, I've included some additional ideas to give you a sense of what kinds of meals and snacks make up a well-proportioned day.

Breakfast
• A bowl of oatmeal with blueberries and sliced strawberries

or

• Low-sugar cereal mix with 1 percent or skim milk and a glass of orange or grapefruit juice

or

• Egg-white omelet filled with onions, tomatoes, mushrooms, and peppers

Lunch
• White-meat turkey or chicken sandwich on whole-grain bread and a cup of tomato-basil soup

or

• Salad with assorted vegetables, canned tuna and low-fat dressing

or

• Teriyaki fish or chicken with brown rice and vegetables

Dinner
• Pasta with chicken and broccoli and a garden salad

or

• Fish with salsa, grilled asparagus, and brown rice

or

• Couscous with curried vegetables and a cup of spinach soup

Snacks

Choose one from this list, twice a day.

• Raw vegetables and fat-free ranch dressing
• Fruit
• One ounce of pretzels
• Air-popped popcorn topped with Worcestershire sauce, vinegar, or cayenne pepper
• Soup (not cream-based)
• A small or medium baked potato topped with salsa
• A small or medium baked sweet potato
• A low-fat frozen yogurt bar
• A frozen fruit bar
• Low-fat or fat-free yogurt with one teaspoon of maple syrup and sliced bananas
• One cup of steamed edamame (see page 81)
• One cup of brown rice
• One ounce of raw walnuts, almonds, or cashews
• One ounce of low-fat cheese
• A low-fat cookie

call "artificial hunger." When you're dehydrated, for example, you may feel as though your body is telling you to eat when all you really need is a glass of water. Similarly, you may crave food when you really need a particular nutrient, such as sodium (the reason tortilla chips might sound particularly good). You can head off these false cravings by making sure that your diet is well balanced and that you're covering all your vitamin and mineral bases. And don't forget about water. You might try having a glass before you snack to see if that alone is enough to satisfy you.

Step 4: Make Healthful Food Choices

Typically, the first thing that people who've decided to lose weight or eat more healthfully think about is what they *can't* eat. How many favorite foods will they have to give up? Will they ever get to eat a luscious dessert again (and, if they do, not feel guilty about it)? It's true that if you hope to drop pounds and change your eating for the better, you probably will have to give up a little of this and a little of that. But I'd prefer that you think about what you *can* eat. There's a world full of flavorful, satisfying foods out there that fit easily into a nutritious, weight-conscious eating plan. You don't have to deprive yourself of foods that you enjoy to reach your goals.

In fact, depriving yourself is probably the *worst* thing you can do. Few people can stick to a diet that denies them any pleasure (at least not for very long!). Or a diet that doesn't provide them with adequate vitamins, minerals, and calories. Whether it's lack of sensory enjoyment or lack of nutrients, something will cause you to crave foods that fall outside your diet's parameters and you'll eventually give in and go back to the (unhealthy) way you ate before.

It might seem strange that so many popular diets have been based on severely limiting your food choices, when clearly that's not the answer. But the problem is, these diets do cause quick weight loss, giving people time to talk them up and recommend them to friends. But come back for a visit later, and see what's happened. Most people quit the diet and gain back the weight. In the short term you may see results, but rigid, restrictive diets are not in your long-term interest.

Human beings were meant to eat a variety of foods. If our bodies were designed to operate like a well-run machine on vitamin C alone, we could live happily on a grapefruit diet. But we get bored psychologically and stretched physiologically—we need the calcium we get from dairy products and dark, leafy greens; the beta-carotene we get from orange-red foods such as squash and tomatoes; and all the other nutrients that are obtained from a varied diet. Far from being weak-willed, someone who can't stay more than a week on the "orange-food-only eating plan" is simply craving foods that will give her body the fuel it needs.

The greater the variety and balance in your diet, the healthier you will be. The more moderately you eat, the greater your chance of losing weight and keeping it off. But I admit that this may take some attitude adjustment on your part. You have to come to the realization that eating healthy food is not a punishment but rather a great gift that you give yourself.

Most of us grew up being rewarded for good behavior with foods that are not particularly good for us. Candy. Cookies. Cake. Chips. The message we got was that foods packed with sugar, salt, and fat are a prize, something to aspire to. Ironically, exercise, which *is* good for us, was a punishment. Anytime you were late for gym class you'd be penalized with a couple of laps around the track or some push-ups. No wonder so many people dislike working out! When you grow up with these messages, you become an adult who values bad food and no exercise. It gets deeply lodged within the psyche. Wouldn't it be wonderful if kids were given healthy foods and exercise as a *reward?* Because, frankly, that's what they are. When you eat well, you are treating yourself to something that will ultimately make you feel good (and, let's be honest, look good, too). Healthy food is a gift.

Some might argue that healthy food is not a gift because it doesn't have the same pleasure factor. I disagree, though I can see why many people think that way. Fat, sugar, and salt add concentrated flavor to food, and it's easy to get accustomed to their intensity. However, other foods, healthy, natural foods—whether they are good-quality fruits and vegetables or lean meats—also have intense flavor. It's just that we've obscured them so long with fat, sugar, and salt that it's hard to remember what they really taste like!

I urge you to rediscover the flavor of *real* food. A deep red, perfectly ripe strawberry. The crunch and pure nutty flavor of an almond. A mouthful of bread made with rich-tasting, chewy whole grains. These are the pleasures you will find if you open yourself up to them. And along the way, you'll discover that you feel good, have more energy for exercise, and achieve a healthier weight. These are great gifts you can give yourself, and all it takes is making some wise food choices.

A Quick Word About Calories

Before you go flipping through the pages of this book looking for the number of calories you should eat, I want to let you know that you won't see it here. It's not that calories don't count; of course they do. To lose weight, you must expend more calories than you take in. It's that simple. But *you* are not that simple. You have a certain frame size, your own specific metabolism, a particular amount of activity that you do each day, and your own individual goals—all of which are probably different from someone else's. One size *doesn't* fit all when it comes to calorie recommendations. I don't even like to suggest a range because it really is just too individual and your energy requirements are always changing. As you get fitter and you raise your metabolism, the number of calories you need per day will probably need to be increased.

How, then, can you know how much you should you eat? There's a good way to judge, and it has to do with how hungry you feel, but first let me explain what you are trying to accomplish. Basically, the amount you eat should fulfill two goals. First, you need to satisfy your nutritional needs. You need to take in enough carbohydrates, fat, protein, vitamins, minerals, and phytochemicals to keep you healthy. That's of number one importance (and is something that many weight loss plans don't take into account).

Your second goal depends on whether you want to lose weight or not. If you want to maintain your weight, you need to eat enough calories to match your body's energy needs: the calories you take in should equal the calories expended. If you want to lose weight, you'll need to eat slightly below your body's energy needs so that you go into calorie debt. It's a delicate balance—getting enough nutrients but not quite enough calories—but it can be done.

If you're trying to maintain your weight, you should eat when you're truly physically hungry and stop before you feel stuffed. If you want to lose fat, you should stop when you feel as if you'd still like to eat a little at the end of a meal—but just a little. That will let you know that your body is warning you it's going to dip into your fat stores, which, again, is what you want to happen.

A life tied to calorie counting is a bore and can really put you off eating healthfully. What I would much rather see you do is get a feel for how much is enough and allow making the right choices to come to you naturally. Ultimately you'll know if you're on the right track by whether your clothes start loosening or not. Remember, the changes you make in your eating behavior are changes you're going to have to live with the rest of your life. This isn't a diet you go onto or off of; it's a way of life, and it should feel as natural to you as breathing. Remember, too, that all the other steps in this book are designed to help you ease into moderate eating. Staying adequately hydrated, getting a grip on emotional eating, exercising, eating breakfast, having an eating cutoff time, redistributing your calories—all these will help you recognize your true physical hunger, which in turn will help you eat moderately.

The Nutrients You Need to Know About

Water's Role in Nutrition

Asked to name nutrients, many people wouldn't put water on the list. But when you consider the definition of a nutrient—a substance that helps the body perform functions that help you stay alive—you can see that water is indeed a nutrient. It also plays an important role in helping you to process other nutrients, from carbohydrates and fat to vitamins and minerals. As I mentioned in Part I, you'll benefit your health by drinking at least eight eight-ounce glasses of water a day. By now you probably know the old trick of using water to fill you up, but water's relation to your weight goes beyond that: every system in your body, including the digestive system, needs water to function. Without adequate hydration, you cannot break down food or metabolize fat efficiently.

You can get water from other sources than just the tap (or a bottle). It's in all beverages and even in foods, particularly fruits and vegetables, which have a high water content. But it's not enough to rely on these sources—particularly if they're beverages that contain caffeine, as caffeine's diuretic effect may cause you to lose some water. Your best bet is still to get those eight glasses of pure, fresh noncarbonated water a day.

The Big Three: Carbohydrates, Fat, and Protein

There has been a lot of guessing going on about what's the best way to divide up your calories each day. My experience has been that there are no perfect numbers but that most people do well with the following percentages. I suggest that you see how they work for you, then fine-tune them as needed. You should try to get approximately:

• 50 to 60 percent of your calories from carbohydrates

• 25 to 30 percent of your calories from fat

• 15 to 20 percent of your calories from protein

Carbohydrates: The Good, the Bad, and the Ugly

When it comes to carbohydrates, the nutrition pendulum has swung back and forth so many times it's enough to make you dizzy. In fact I think a lot of people do find the whole matter of carbohydrates dizzying. Are they in? Are they out? Which are good? Which are bad? Do they make you fat? Can they help you lose weight?

Let's start by defining what carbohydrates are. In the big picture, they are a major source of energy for the body and the primary source of fuel for the brain. In the smaller picture, carbohydrates are nutrients made of a combination of carbon, hydrogen, and oxygen molecules. Linked together in units, these elements make different kinds of carbohydrates, depending on the number of units. Sugars, such as sucrose (table sugar), glucose, fructose (the sugar in fruit), maltose, lactose (milk sugar), and galactose—also known as simple carbohydrates—are made of one or two units. Starches and fiber—complex carbohydrates—are made of many more units.

Carbohydrates (except for fiber) are broken down by your digestive system and converted into the single-unit sugar glucose, also known as blood sugar. Some of the glucose is converted into glycogen, a form of carbohydrate that is stored in the muscles and liver; some is used immediately for energy. And if you take in more carbohydrate calories than your body needs, the excess glucose will be converted to and stored as body fat.

For a long time, people thought that starchy foods were fattening. Then suddenly experts started encouraging dieters to eat foods such as pasta, bread, and rice. Since carbohydrates have only 4 calories per gram as compared to fat, which has 9 calories per gram, they reasoned that starchy carbohydrates really weren't fattening after all! What they didn't count on was that some people would start piling their plates high with spaghetti and eating practically a whole baguette before their main course ever got to them. Gram for gram, starchy carbohydrates aren't overly caloric, but those grams (and calories) can add up. If you eat portions of starchy carbohydrates above and beyond your calorie needs, then yes, you will put on weight.

When people started to realize that they weren't losing weight on high-carbohydrate diets, the pendulum swung way back the other way and carbohydrates became dietary bad guys again. The truth, as always, is somewhere in the middle. Some carbohydrates are better than others, and, like any food, they have to be eaten in moderation. In order to

What's One Serving?

You don't have to measure your food to know what a proper serving is. One-half cup is about the size of your fist; 3 ounces is as large as a deck of playing cards; 1 ounce is approximately the size of your thumb.

Fruit
- 1 medium apple, banana, or orange
- ½ grapefruit, mango, or papaya
- ½ cup berries or grapes
- ¾ cup juice
- ¼ cup dried fruit

Vegetables
- ½ cup chopped nonleafy, raw vegetables such as green pepper, zucchini, or carrots
- 1 cup leafy, raw vegetables such as lettuce, spinach, or Swiss chard
- ½ cup cooked vegetables such as broccoli, green beans, or squash
- 1 small baked potato
- ¾ cup vegetable (such as tomato or carrot) juice
- Lettuce, tomato and onion (on a sandwich)

Grains
- 1 slice whole-grain bread
- ½ bagel or English muffin
- 1 6-inch tortilla
- ½ cup cooked rice, pasta, or barley
- ½ cup cooked oatmeal
- ¾ cup ready-to-eat cereal

Meat, Poultry, Seafood, and Other Protein Foods
- 2 to 3 ounces cooked meat, poultry or fish
- 2 to 3 ounces canned tuna or salmon
- 1 egg

- 2 tablespoons nut butter
- 4 ounces tofu
- ½ cup cooked lentils, peas or dry beans

Dairy
- 1 cup milk or yogurt
- 1½ ounces cheese such as cheddar or mozzarella
- ½ cup ricotta or cottage cheese

make healthy choices, I think it will help if you understand the differences among carbohydrate foods and why some are better choices than others. Let's start with the best of the bunch.

✓ Fruits and Vegetables

Eat at least two servings of fruit and four servings of vegetables each day.

People tend to forget that fruits and vegetables are primarily carbohydrates, but in fact they're your best carbohydrate picks. This is not just because they're an excellent source of the vitamins and minerals that you need to keep your body operating properly but because they contain micronutrients such as phytochemicals and antioxidants, which can actually prevent disease. The research linking a high intake of fruits and vegetables to a lowered risk of several forms of cancer is just too strong to ignore. One of the healthiest things you can do is to bolster your diet with plenty of produce.

This is also a good idea from a weight loss perspective. Fruits and vegetables are satisfying without being calorie dense. For the most part, you can fill up on them without fear of adding body fat.

Different health organizations have different recommendations about the number of fruit and vegetable servings you should eat daily, but no one suggests going lower than a total of five servings a day. I'm going to ask you to eat more—at least two servings of fruits and four servings of vegetables each day. If you'd like to eat three pieces of fruit a day, go for it. But you really don't need more than that if you're trying to lose weight; you'll just end up with excess calories.

In regards to vegetables, I just want to add that, contrary to what is often said, you don't have to skip potatoes even if you're trying to lose weight. Of course, I'm not talking about French fries (the most widely consumed vegetable, in the United States). I'm referring to regular potatoes, which, even though they are starchy, can be a good addition to a healthy diet (see more on this in "What's the Glycemic Index?" on page 66). Especially sweet potatoes! They are just packed with the antioxidant beta-carotene and other nutrients.

✓ Whole Grains

Eat 7 servings each day.

You might notice that I say *whole* grains. This is an important distinction. Whole grains have not been processed, so all their parts are intact, including the bran (outer coating) and the germ. These are the parts of the grain that are rich in B vitamins, trace minerals, and fiber, as well as disease-fighting antioxidants. Many manufacturers of processed grain products fortify their foods, putting the vitamins and minerals stripped away in the processing back in. But eating one of these products is not the same as eating a whole-grain food: the manufacturers don't put everything back; the only way to get all the nutrients is to eat the whole grain.

Plus, there's no replacement for fiber. The body doesn't digest fiber, but it plays a significant role in good health. One of its most important benefits is that it helps remove waste products from the body so that the digestive system has minimal contact with toxins. One kind of fiber—the insoluble kind found in whole oats or oat bran—can also help lower cholesterol levels. Fiber can help with weight loss, too. Fiber gives foods bulk so that they fill you up on relatively few calories.

If you're used to eating white bread, white rice, regular semolina pastas, and foods made with white flour, you might find the taste and texture of whole grains a little rough at first. But trust me, you will come to enjoy them as you make the switch. In many cases, these product actually have more flavor than their stripped-down counterparts. Start slowly, substituting one whole-grain product for its refined counterpart at a time, but also keep in mind that if you prepare them well and pair them with other good foods, they'll be easier for you to accept. That's one of my goals in providing you with great recipes—the dishes at the back of this book will go a long way toward helping you grow to like whole grains.

✓ Refined Sugar

Eat only occasionally.

Refined sugar (or table sugar) falls into the category of simple carbohydrates. And that's exactly what's wrong with it: it's simple—you don't get much else with it. No vitamins and minerals, no fiber. Refined sugar really contributes nothing to your diet—except, of course, calories. If you eat a lot of sugar at the expense of more nutritious foods, your health is really going to suffer because you're probably not going to get the vitamins, minerals, and fiber you need. And if you eat a lot of sugar on top of more nutritious foods, you'll probably get too many calories. Either way, you're going to lose: there is solid evidence linking a high intake of refined sugar to obesity and an increased risk of diabetes and other diseases.

Typically we think of refined sugar as table sugar, but it also comes in other forms. The most common is corn syrup, the main ingredient in most soft drinks and many other sweet commercial foods. The word "corn" in its name may make you think that corn syrup is healthier than sugar, but it's not healthy in the least. It may even be worse than sugar. Fructose is a slightly better simple sugar that's also used to sweeten many processed foods, but the best way to eat fructose is in fruit. You just can't beat fruit for sweetness combined with good nutrition—it's a perfect little package.

Eliminating sugar from your diet completely is a noble goal, although a difficult one and not entirely necessary. You can still have some refined sugar in your diet and be healthy, but try to have it mostly in foods that you make yourself; that way you can control how much you use. The dessert recipes in this book, for instance, use some sugar but in very moderate portions.

If you have a sweet tooth, fruit can also really help you cut back on refined sugar. Good fruit, that is. One way I define good fruit is fruit that is in season. When you buy a peach in January, chances are that it was grown somewhere far away where it's warm during our winter, then transported to your local grocery store. But fruit that must survive transit is picked early—too early for it to sweeten on the vine—so it will never taste truly delicious by the time it gets to you. Try to buy fruit in season; it's even better if you can get it from a farmers' market, since that fruit is typically left on the vine to sweeten till the last minute, then picked just before being brought to market.

What's the Glycemic Index? (And How Much Does It Matter?)

If you haven't heard of the glycemic index, you probably will at some time or another. Many people are trying to live by its rules, while others are simply confused by what it means and how it should affect their choice of carbohydrates. In brief, the glycemic index is a measure of how quickly carbohydrates are converted to glucose and how quickly your blood sugar rises as a result. When blood sugar rises rapidly, it causes a corresponding surge in insulin, and insulin, in turn, attempts to lower the amount of blood sugar by moving it into your cells and encouraging the deposition of body fat.

You can see why it's to your disadvantage to eat foods that rate high on the glycemic index—that is, foods that promote a spike in blood sugar or insulin. The foods that are highest on the index include white bread, sugar, carrots, corn and cornflakes, brown and white rice, and baked potatoes. I'd like to see you eliminate some of the foods with little nutritional value, such as white bread, white rice, and sugar from

Remember:

Eat in moderation:
- Fruit (2 or 3 servings per day)
- Vegetables (5 to 8 servings per day)
- Whole grains (brown rice, whole-grain breads, whole-grain pastas, whole-grain cereals, oats) (7 servings per day)

Limit:
- Processed-grain foods (pastas made with refined flour, white rice, white bread)
- Table sugar
- Sugary cereals
- Soda
- Candy
- Cake
- Pie
- White-flour foods

your diet, but certain other foods high on the index are perfectly healthy. One of the pitfalls of the glycemic index is that some nutritious foods inadvertently get a bad rap. There are a few reasons why.

First of all, because of the way the scale measures food, many vegetables come in high, but it would take about twelve servings of carrots, four potatoes, or three cups of corn to match the blood glucose effects of a candy bar. You're probably not going to eat that many vegetables in one sitting, so in this case it's a waste of time and energy to worry about it. It would be a shame to leave these nutritious foods out of your diet for the wrong reasons.

Another problem with the glycemic index is that it doesn't take into account what happens when you eat several foods together, as you generally do at a meal. Fat, for instance, blunts the blood sugar–raising effects of other foods because it slows down digestion, as do acidic foods such as lemon and orange juice and vinegar. If you have a bowl-ful of cornflakes with low-fat milk and a glass of orange juice (as opposed to, say, eating cornflakes by the handful), your blood sugar will rise at a much more moderate rate. Fiber and protein are food components that diminish the glycemic response. Oats and other whole grains, beans, basmati rice (which is better than processed white rice), fruits (in particular, apples, berries, and cherries), and vegetables are all good choices if you're hoping to avoid an insulin spike.

The only time I would recommend that you keep the glycemic index in mind is when you're snacking and are therefore more likely to eat a single food at a time. (The University of Sydney, which sponsors a Web site that gives the glycemic ratings of different foods, is a good place to learn more about the subject; see www.glycemicindex.com.) Also bear in mind that the larger the meal you eat, the more rapidly your blood sugar will rise and the greater the chance that you'll have an insulin spike. As I discussed in Step 3, distributing your calories evenly throughout the day has numerous health benefits, and avoiding an insulin spike is among them.

The Skinny on Fat

When it comes to dietary fat, people generally have two ways of thinking. They're either fat-phobic and try to exist mainly on fat-free foods, or they know fat is bad for them but they feel that food just isn't worthwhile without it. And I mean without a *lot* of it. As with the carbohydrate dilemma, the best way to deal with fat is somewhere in between.

You need fat in your diet. It helps you digest food, creates hormones, transports nutrients, and increases your immunity to disease. It also makes you feel full after you eat. And of course, fat tastes good, sometimes just on its own, but mostly because it enhances the flavor of other foods. Can you imagine lettuce without dressing? That's probably not going to do it for you. Sure, you can find happiness with a fat-free dressing, but even just a little bit of fat can make a world of difference. (If you've ever compared fat-free cream cheese to the low-fat kind, you know what I'm talking about.)

All this said, there are also some reasonable concerns about dietary fat. What first pops in to the mind of anyone trying to lose weight is that fats are, well, fattening. Fat has 9 calories per gram, more than twice the amount that carbohydrates and protein do. You get a lot of energy—but not a lot of nutrition—from something like a tablespoon of oil. Above and beyond that, a high fat intake is associated with a greater risk of heart disease and other illnesses. Yes, you need some fat in your diet, but there's little reason to make it more than 30 percent of your total daily calories. And it is important to be aware of what kinds of fats you are consuming. All fats are definitely not created equal.

Fats are composed of a mix of glycerol and something called fatty acids. It's the fatty acids that determine how healthy or unhealthy a fat is. "Bad" fats—that is, those that have been shown to raise blood cholesterol levels—are those with a high percentage of saturated fatty acids (saturated fats) or *trans*–fatty acids (*trans*-fats). Saturated fats include fats from animal foods, such as meat, poultry, butter, ice cream, milk, lard, and chicken fat, as well as palm and coconut oils. *Trans*-fats are hydrogenated fats—fats that have been altered with a hydrogen molecule to make them stable and solid at room temperature. Margarine and vegetable shortening are *trans*-fats. You may also see them on ingredient listings under the name partially hydrogenated oil.

Unless you eat no animal foods, it's hard to completely avoid bad fats, but I recommend limiting them as much as possible. There is another class of fats called polyunsaturated fats, which include safflower oil, corn oil, and sunflower oil. I'd limit them as much as possible, too.

Instead, choose "good" fats—those that may raise HDL, or "good" cholesterol levels. These fats are high in monounsaturated fatty acids and include olive oil, canola oil, and avocado. There's quite a bit of research showing that olive oil is the best type of fat going; I suggest making it your cooking oil of choice. I myself make everything with olive oil, even omelets. Depending on your own personal preference, you can buy olive oils that range in flavor from light (you can hardly tell they're olive oil) to hearty extra-virgin varieties.

There is one other healthy kind of fat, called omega-3 fatty acids, of which you should be aware. Research shows that these fats can help prevent heart attacks, and there are ongoing studies looking at whether they may protect against everything from Parkinson's disease to Alzheimer's disease—they may even turn out to have health-preserving powers beyond what we now suspect. To get omega-3s, it helps if you like fish as they're most abundant in fatty fishes such as mackerel, herring, sardines, albacore tuna, and salmon (two servings of fish a week is the recommended dose to lower the risk of heart attack). If you're not a fish eater or are concerned about toxins in fish, there is another route you can try: your body can also convert flaxseed, canola, and soybean oils into omega-3s. Purslane, a vegetable used in Mexican and Mediterranean dishes, is another good vegetarian source.

Your best approach to reducing the fat in your diet is to use common sense. Start by cutting out foods that are especially high in fat, such as fatty cuts of beef and highly processed lunch meats such as salami and bologna. Nix the cream sauces and potato and tortilla chips. Hold the butter. Choose low-fat or skim dairy products and salad dressings that have moderate amounts of oil. (Better yet, make your own; see any of the dressing recipes in this book.)

I particularly urge you to forgo fried foods, especially those made in restaurants. Commercially made fried foods are often cooked in oil that is used over and over again. This reuse can produce harmful by-products, adding to the damage the fat (often saturated) can do. If you must have the occasional fried food treat, make it at home.

The Truth About Protein

The question on everybody's lips these days seems to be "How much protein should I eat?" I wish I had a pat answer, but the truth is that how much protein you need is a very individual issue. For most people, protein should make up somewhere between 15 and 20 percent of their total calories, but some people need a little more. I recommend the trial-and-error approach—see how you feel in general and when you're exercising. If you're eating too much protein at the expense of carbohydrates and fat—the main sources of fuel for exercise—you're bound to feel it. You really need a fairly high intake of carbohydrates to fuel exercise, a fact that's often overlooked. Books about high-protein diets don't talk much about exercise, because these diets are not optimal for exercisers.

Many of the diets that are so popular today recommend quite a bit more protein than 15 to 20 percent. While I talked in the introduction about why those diets are self-defeating, I just want to reiterate that they have the potential to cause some health concerns. If you rely too heavily on protein at the expense of other nutrients, you may place added stress on your kidneys and liver. In addition, if it is deprived of carbohydrate and fat, your body will break down its muscles for energy, ultimately limiting the amount of calories you burn (muscle requires a lot of energy to maintain, and the more you have of it, the more calories you burn). Another side effect is that when it is denied carbohydrate, the body cannot burn fat efficiently. Fat, as it's often said, burns in a carbohydrate flame. Then there are those other nasty effects of a high-protein diet, such as gas, bad breath, and clouded thinking.

When you eat an overabundance of protein, you will likely lose some weight, but much of it will be water weight and it ultimately won't stay off when you go back to eating normally (which you eventually will because a high-protein diet is so unimaginative that you'll get sick of it after a while). Much of that water comes from your muscles, which hold water along with glycogen. When they use the glycogen for energy (and since you're not eating much carbohydrate, none comes in to replace it), they release the water and you weigh less. However, as soon as you begin eating carbohydrates again, your muscles will sock away more glycogen—and with it, water. The water weight you lost will return.

Protein, *in moderation,* is essential for good health. It's made of up several different amino acids, nine of which are essential for building, maintaining, and repairing body tissues. And that includes muscle tissue. If you hope to make gains from your strength training exercises, you'll need adequate protein in your diet. Your body's production of hormones and antibodies depends on protein as well.

Protein comes in both animal and vegetarian forms. Animal sources—meat, poultry, fish, eggs, dairy products—contain all nine of the essential amino acids. Vegetarian sources—nuts, seeds, legumes, and, in smaller amounts, whole grains and some vegetables—are lacking one or more of the essential nine, except for soy and quinoa which are complete. If you don't eat animal foods, your body will combine the amino acids from different plant foods that you eat. But for it to do so, you need to eat a variety of plant protein sources throughout the day. You don't, however, have to combine specific foods at one meal; that idea has been disproven.

The key to meeting your protein needs adequately is finding high-quality sources that are not coupled with saturated fat. Fish, eggs, lean cuts of meat and poultry, soy in the form of miso, tofu, or tempeh, legumes, and nuts all fit the bill. The inclusion of eggs might surprise you, but although they've been much maligned in the past, eggs and in particular egg whites are a great source of protein. I do, however, suggest that you balance your animal sources of protein with vegetarian sources—studies link diets high in animal foods with an increased risk of cancer.

Other Considerations

✓ Alcohol

I hope you won't peg me as a Puritan when I say that I'd like you to limit your alcohol intake, if not eliminate it altogether. Although I like a glass of wine or a beer as much as the next person, I can't help but be aware of all the negative aspects of drinking. And it can really put a crimp in your plans to lose or even just maintain your weight.

For one thing, at 7 calories per gram, alcohol has more calories than carbohydrates and protein (4 calories per gram each) and only slightly less than fat (9 calories per gram). Perhaps worse is the fact that it slows the metabolism, and the effect can linger for days. And, of course, as you drink alcohol you become more uninhibited, and often, so does your eating. It's hard to keep to your commitment to eating well when you're not thinking straight. It's often also harder to exercise the day after you've been drinking, so it's really a triple whammy: your metabolism slows down, you eat poorly, and you don't work out as vigorously. Ultimately, you'll take in more calories and burn fewer of them.

Alcohol does have redeeming qualities for some individuals. There is, for instance, some evidence to suggest that red wine thins the blood, helping to prevent heart attack. But there are also other ways to get the same effect. Each day, I personally take two children's aspirins. They thin the blood and may also guard against colon and esophageal cancers. Wines have antioxidants, but so do many other foods (such as grapes), and if you're trying to lose weight, they may be a better choice. Remember, all the exercise you're doing will help your heart, too.

A good way to start cutting down on alcohol is to estimate how much you drink, then cut it in half. And try to only have one drink at a sitting. It's the first one that tastes the best anyway, isn't it? You'll notice that several of the recipes in this book give you the option of adding alcohol. Keep in mind that when alcohol is brought to a boil it evaporates, essentially eliminating the negative effects while preserving the flavor.

✓ Supplements

Invariably when I have a public speaking engagement, someone (and sometimes many people) will ask me what I think of some kind of "miracle" supplement that they've heard about. It might be one of those pills that promise to burn fat or increase your metabolism or one that guarantees muscle growth. I generally tell them that I put these in the "don't bother" category, as in don't bother wasting your time or your money. There are no miracles; no pill is going to do it all for you.

There are, however, supplements that I do believe can help improve your nutritional status and provide good insurance against nutrient deficits. They are a good addition to a healthy diet; *food* should still be your number one source of nutrition. There simply is no replacement for a healthy diet, especially one that's high in fruits and vegetables. It seems that we learn something new about how produce improves our well-being every other day, and we haven't even begun to scratch the surface.

While ideally you'd get all the nutrients you need from food, the reality is that it's difficult to get a high enough dosage of some of the vitamins, minerals, and antioxidants that we know can help prevent disease. When you do supplement your diet, it's important to keep in mind that you also get nutrients from other sources, so be careful not to accidentally megadose. These days, many foods and beverages are fortified with vitamins and minerals, so if you're not checking food labels, you may be getting more than you bargained for. I personally supplement in the low end of the recommended dosages and eat healthful, balanced meals. It usually all adds up to just the right amount.

I prefer single-nutrient supplements to multivitamins mainly because they give you more control over the dosages you're taking. Multivitamins can be so varied that they can make it a challenge to get the doses of the specific nutrients that you want. With singles you have more control. Here are the supplements that I take daily and that, if they fit into your diet, you may want to try, too.

- Vitamin C: 100 to 200 milligrams
- B complex: Make sure that it contains 400 micrograms of folic acid; the other B vitamins in the complex will vary, but should be something like this: 10 milligrams of thiamin; 10 milligrams of

riboflavin; 50 milligrams of pantothenic acid; 10 milligrams of vitamin B6; 10 micrograms of vitamin B12
- Vitamin E: 400 to 800 International Units (make sure it's natural d-alpha tocopherol)
- Selenium: 200 micrograms
- Beta-carotene: 25,000 IU; if possible, get a carotenoid complex that contains this amount of beta-carotene as well as other carotenoids

If you're over the age of forty (to help prevent osteoporosis):

- Vitamin D: 400 IU
- Calcium: 1,000 milligram

Creating a Healthy Kitchen

A client once invited me to look into her refrigerator and cabinets to see if I could make some suggestions about how she could change her eating habits. I took a look around her kitchen, and it was full, very full of food—but there was hardly a thing to eat. Well, there were things you *could* eat; however, there were very few items that I would have recommended that she *should* eat. Most of the foods were highly processed, and many of them were high in sugar, fat, and preservatives. All the grain products were refined (not a whole kernel in the bunch), and she could have done a lot better in the cooking and salad oils department. There wasn't a bottle of olive oil in sight.

Over time, as I surveyed other clients' kitchens, I discovered that many people's pantries are stocked with foods that are sadly lacking in nutritional value. Sometimes they try to justify these items, saying that they just bought them that one time or that they were for someone else in the household, but those excuses don't negate the damage the unhealthy foods can do. If you know it's not nutritious, simply don't put it into your grocery cart.

Having healthy foods on hand in your kitchen is half the battle. It's kind of like building a house: if you want a sturdy, well-built home, you need to use good materials. Likewise, if you want to build healthful meals, you need the right ingredients. As part of your commitment to this program, I urge you to survey your own kitchen and consider tossing out some of the products that will impede your progress toward weight loss and good health.

Start with the oils. I personally don't think you need to use anything other than olive oil, except perhaps for some kinds of baking. Olive oil is the best for your health, and it comes in a range of flavor intensities. (I personally love the strong taste of extra-virgin olive oil.) If you need another oil for baking, choose canola. Get rid of the polyunsaturates (safflower, peanut, and corn oils) as well as the saturated fats (lard and chicken fat) and *trans*-fats (margarine, hydrogenated oils, shortening).

Next, attack the refined sugar in your cupboards, beginning with soda. Soda, a mix of sugar, water, and artificial flavor, contributes significantly to obesity in this country and, in particular, the obesity of children. And while we're on the subject of beverages, take note that juice is another high-sugar drink. While it's true that the sugar in juice is natural fructose and that, unlike sodas, most juices come with some vitamins and minerals, all that sugar adds up to a substantial number of calories. More than a small glass at breakfast is too much if you're trying to lose weight. And not all juices are created equal. Apple juice really doesn't have nearly as much to offer as citrus juices, and some juices, such as cranberry, are often sweetened with sugar or corn syrup. When you're buying juices, you really need to read the labels closely. I'll talk more about this a little bit later.

Water is always a great choice, but on those occasions that you want something with more kick to it, you might try one of the many new fruit-flavored noncarbonated waters. Many of these are also fortified with vitamins, and I think they're a promising alternative to sugary and diet soft drinks. The best ones are made from purified water and have a shot of different vitamins, a bit of flavor, and a small amount of fructose (to mask the vitamin's bitterness). They don't have many calories and can help you keep all your nutrient bases covered. If you prefer a low-calorie or noncaloric drink, there are now also noncarbonated fruit-flavored waters *without* vitamins on the market. Either option can help you cut down on unwanted sugar.

Once the soda is gone, dump all the refined-sugar sweets (cookies, pastries, even granola bars), too—including things you don't think of as sweets but really are, such as high-sugar cereals and jams. Replace them with similar foods that are sugar-free or fruit-sweetened. You may want to use *some* refined sugar in cooking—in fact, some of the recipes here call for it. But using it in your *own* cooking, which allows you to control how much you use, is a lot better than buying foods that contain sugar—manufacturers simply add too much.

I also suggest that you get rid of white bread and other baked goods made with refined white flour and replace them with whole-grain versions. This might mean, for instance, switching from white wheat crackers to European whole-grain crackers. Or swapping white rice for brown or wild rice and refined hot cereals such as Cream of Wheat for whole-grain ones such as Wheatena or oatmeal. Really be vigilant with your ready-to-eat cereals, too. You may think that some of them are whole-grain because they seem, well, grainy; but they may just be processed to look that way.

If, like most people, you've been eating refined-grain products such as white bread, white rice, and conventional pasta for years, switching to whole grains might be tough at first. You might start with whole-wheat bread—it's fairly easy to get used to—then gradually add some other whole-grain foods to your diet. The added health benefits these foods provide will be worth any initial struggle you have with them, and I feel certain that eventually you will begin to enjoy them.

Fatty, processed meats such as salami and bologna, as well as full-fat dairy products, will not benefit your body. Buy lean cold cuts and low-fat or nonfat dairy products. Low-fat and skim milk, nonfat yogurt, and low-fat cottage cheese and hard cheeses are good examples of reduced-fat foods that are quite healthy. They provide numerous nutrients, and nothing has been added back to them to make up for the fat that was taken out. But not all low-fat and fat-free foods are formulated as conscientiously. Some manufacturers of fat-free foods replace the fat with sugar, so that ultimately they're not really healthier and may have just as many calories as their fat-containing counterparts. Sometimes they have even more.

If you've never been a reader of the fine print on labels, you'll need to start if you hope to take home the healthiest foods from the supermarket. Look at the nutrition information provided on the label for fat, fiber, and calorie counts, keeping in mind the portion size. What may look like one serving to you, may be *two* (or more!) servings in the manufacturer's mind. For instance, a serving of cereal is usually defined by the manufacturer as three quarters of a cup. If you have big cereal bowls, you may be pouring in a cup and a half, while at the same time thinking that the calorie count on the box applies to your bowlful.

Also, check the ingredients list; that's where you'll really find the lowdown on what you're getting. The first ingredient on the list is contained in the largest amount, and the list descends from there. If sugar (or corn syrup) is the first ingredient, it's not a product you want. If sugar is way down on the list and healthier ingredients such as whole-grain flour are first, it's a better choice.

Like any major lifestyle change, restocking your kitchen should be a gradual process. Throw out the unhealthy foods in your kitchen (or at least don't replace them as you use them) as you feel emotionally ready to give them up. The change isn't going to "take" if you're unprepared to make it. Realize, too, that working on your diet is an ongoing endeavor. I'm still fine-tuning my own diet, and I will for the rest of my life.

When you are ready to make changes, try the nutritious replacements I mentioned one or two at a time (the recipes in this book will also help you) and give yourself a chance to get used to them. I think that over time you'll find that, healthy foods are fresher and more intensely flavored than their unhealthy counterparts.

Eight Great Choices

One of the most important things you can do for your health is to eat a varied diet. Because each food you eat contains a unique assortment of nutrients, the more diverse your diet, the more nutrients you'll end up getting. Variety keeps eating interesting, too. Your meals are likely to be more satisfying if you haven't eaten the same thing the day before (and the day before that).

Within a varied diet, there's some room for liberal use of what I like to think of as superfoods. Some of these foods are nutrition powerhouses—that is, ounce for ounce they contain more vitamins, minerals, and phytochemicals than other foods. Some of them are simply healthy and either bring hard-to-get nutrients to the table or, because of their taste and texture, provide a great substitute for less nutritious choices. Some of them are even foods that you may have written off as unhealthy and will be surprised to find that they can be part of a nutritious diet. Many of the recipes in this book include these superfoods, so you'll have a chance to get to know them through your own home cooking. Here are eight great ones to look for.

Olive Oil

As I said earlier, I use olive oil for just about everything, even for making foods such as omelets, which are usually cooked in butter or margarine. Olive oil has significant health benefits. It's been shown to lower total blood cholesterol levels without lowering HDL (good cholesterol) levels, and it may even raise HDL levels. And it's a good source of carotenoids and antioxidants, including vitamin E, an antioxidant that appears to help prevent heart disease.

Shopping for a bottle of olive oil these days is a little like shopping for wine. There are many varieties and estate-produced bottles, and the prices can range from a few bucks to upward of $20. Typically, the more you pay, the purer the flavor, but there are some great-tasting olive oils around (such as Bertolli) that can be found in supermarkets and are of high quality. I generally keep a couple of olive oils on hand. The one I use most often is an extra-virgin olive oil. Extra-virgin means that the oil has been cold-pressed without chemicals (other oils are sometimes extracted through the use of solvents). It's the fruitiest of the oils and adds wonderful flavor to food. In fact, you really need to use only small amounts of the darker extra-virgin oils—the flavor is so intense that a little dab will do you—and that will help you keep your calorie intake down.

I also keep a light olive oil around. It has very little olivey flavor and is good for dishes where you want other flavors to shine. Light olive oil, for instance, works well in Asian stir-fries because it doesn't overpower (or clash with) other flavors you might use, such as sesame, ginger, and rice wine vinegar. In an Indian dish, light olive oil can be substituted for the staple ghee (clarified butter) without obscuring the cumin and curry flavorings.

Soy

Reducing your intake of animal foods is a good idea: people whose diets are abundant in animal foods have a higher risk of cancer. Soy is a great substitute for animal protein, and it has some health benefits of its own. Studies have shown that an ingredient in soy called isoflavones decreases the risk of heart disease, and there's ongoing research looking at the link between soy and cancer reduction.

Tofu—soybean curd—is the most commonly eaten form of soy, though a lot of people don't like the taste of it; it's too bland, they say. But that's exactly what's great about it: it takes on the taste of anything you cook it with. Be creative about the sauces and other foods with which you pair tofu, because it will sop those flavors right up and taste delicious. If you haven't tried it, I urge you to give the Tofu and Broccoli Stir-Fry on page 162 a shot. Alternatively, you can now also find soybeans still in the pod (known as edamame) in many markets, both fresh and frozen. To cook them, you simply place them in boiling water for 5 minutes, drain, and place in a bowl. If you like, sprinkle them lightly with salt, then pop them out of the shell and into your mouth. Edamame are also great thrown into salads and mixed into stir-fries and rice dishes.

Mushrooms

Many people think that mushrooms don't have any nutrients. I don't know how that myth got started, but mushrooms are actually a good source of the antioxidant selenium as well as potassium and B vitamins. So, no, they're not nutritionally empty, and while they're low in calories, they're exceptionally filling. In fact, mushrooms are one of my favorite foods. I use them in sandwiches, in soups, and sautéed with a little olive oil and garlic as a side dish. Mushrooms' meaty texture makes them a good substitute for meat; portabellas, in particular, do a pretty good imitation of steak. If you're used to eating just button mushrooms, try to expand your mushroom horizons. Shitakes, morels, and oyster, porcini, and crimini mushrooms all have their own unique texture and taste. You'll have an opportunity to try them out in the recipes on pages 122 and 197.

Walnuts, Almonds, and Nut Butters

In the past, I've advised people to limit their intake of nuts and nut butters. But now so much research has confirmed that nuts provide a healthy form of protein and fat that I've revised my thinking on the matter. Although they should be eaten in moderation—they are still somewhat caloric—I recommend them as part of a healthy diet.

Nuts are especially good as snacks. When you eat a small handful of walnuts or almonds, your hunger will probably vanish—the fat and the intensity of the nuts' natural flavor makes them very satisfying. Just a thin spread of an almond, cashew, or macadamia nut butter (my top choices for nut butters) on a slice of whole-grain bread is very filling. Nuts—almonds in particular—are also good sources of fiber and protein. I like to sprinkle nuts on vegetable and fruit salads to add a little protein to them. Of course, as I said, I wouldn't recommend setting a whole bowlful of nuts in front of you and going at it. But in moderation, they can help you get some important nutrients and keep your hunger in check.

Eggs

People are often surprised to hear me recommend eggs since they've been a health pariah for so long. But we now know a lot more about the cholesterol in foods than we did just a few years ago. While anyone who has high blood cholesterol levels still has to watch his or her dietary cholesterol intake (and we all should eat foods containing cholesterol in moderation), it turns out that the cholesterol in foods does not do as much damage as we once thought. Of greater risk to your arteries are *trans*-fats, such as hydrogenated oils.

Now some foods, such as eggs, are back on the good-for-you list. (It's almost like what happened in the Woody Allen movie *Sleeper,* when Woody's character awakens to find that deep-fat fries and hot fudge are known for their health-giving properties.) The news about eggs is good news as far as I'm concerned. They're great little packages of nutrients and exceptionally high-quality protein.

If you're prone to high blood cholesterol, you may want to stick more to egg whites than to whole eggs, but don't worry, you're not being shorted: egg whites are an excellent source of high-quality protein. If you're not inclined to give up the yolks completely, you can lower the number you use. Scramble one whole egg and two egg whites, for example, or, when a recipe calls for several eggs, replace one or two of them with extra egg whites (1 egg = 2 egg whites). That way you'll get the flavor of the yolk but not as much cholesterol.

Whenever possible, opt for organic eggs or those from free-range chickens. Ideally and if you can find them, buy organic eggs that come from free-range chickens. Growers who put extra effort into the feeding and care of their chickens produce more nutritious eggs, without traces of hormones or antibiotics. (For the same reasons, it's also a good idea to buy organic and/or free-range poultry whenever possible.) Some producers are now offering omega-3 eggs, produced by chickens that are fed grain rich in heart-healthy omega-3 fatty acids.

Leafy Greens

The days when salads were primarily made from torn iceberg lettuce are gone. Or at least they should be! Iceberg doesn't have much to offer in the way of vitamins and minerals, but darker greens do. Make your salads from mixes of romaine, watercress, spinach, arugula, purslane, mesclun mix, and other dark greens. For cooked dishes, try greens such as kale, chard, and mustard, collard, and beet greens. The latter (broccoli falls into this category, too) are rich in beta-carotene and one of the few good vegetarian sources of calcium. They make easy side dishes (just sauté with a little olive oil and garlic), but if you're a little wary of their bold flavor, chop some up and throw it into a tomato sauce, then serve over pasta. You'll hardly notice the greens, but you'll get all the nutrients they have to offer.

Foods Rich in Omega-3 Fatty Acids

Omega-3 fatty acids are found in fish, especially fish from cold waters. Mackerel, bluefish, sardines, herring, tuna, and salmon have the highest concentrations. While I believe in including fish in a well-balanced diet, I am concerned about the quality of our coastal waters, lakes, and streams. Heavy metals and other toxins are increasingly found within fish (as well as other animals). If this trend continues, we will all be replacing fish with healthier choices. You can also get omega-3s from flaxseed, which can be sprinkled onto cereal or (in oil form) mixed into smoothies. Purslane and canola and soybean oil are also sources.

Berries

One easy and delicious way to get antioxidants into your diet is to eat berries—blueberries, blackberries, cranberries, strawberries, and raspberries. Gram for gram, they have more antioxidants than any other type of fruit. I like them because they're so flavorful (that is, the ones that are bought in season are) and they're easy to toss on top of cereal or nibble on for a snack. Berries also make the perfect ending to a nice meal. They have an elegance and lusciousness that make them a standout (and easy-to-make) dessert.

Where to Shop for Good Food

Grocery shopping is one of those activities that many people do on autopilot. You find a store you like—or one that is convenient—and you travel the same aisles over and over, often throwing the same old foods into your cart. As you begin to change your eating habits, you'll need to change your shopping habits, too. This might mean exploring new stores or even just looking at your usual market with a fresh eye.

I know from my travels around the country that some cities, towns, and suburbs have their choice of markets vying for the dollars of health-conscious shoppers. They're stocked with gorgeous produce and nutritious staples and sometimes even have healthy take-out food. However, other communities have none, or almost none, of these wonderful places to shop. Instead, they're serviced solely by stores that carry almost no healthy snacks, whole grains, fresh fish, or interesting condiments. Even if you're committed to increasing your fruit and vegetable intake, these markets' drab produce sections can make it really hard to stay motivated.

But I see improvements happening quickly. A few years ago, I visited a town in the Midwest where you couldn't find a decent piece of fruit if you spent the whole day looking. Recently, I went back to the same town, this time at the invitation of the owner of a beautiful new grocery store stocked with all kinds of nutritious offerings, including a whole section of organic produce. The owner, a man who's passionate about healthy food himself, had listened to what people in his town were saying and found that others cared about good food, too. His response was to open this great store—a perfect example of demand bringing about change. It pays to ask for good food to be sold in your area.

No matter where you live or what options are available to you, it's important to be able to find healthy foods where you shop. The following is a list of markets and other food purveyors, some of which are admittedly better than others, but all of which can help you eat nutritiously if you navigate them properly.

Farmers' Markets

I always thought the ideal way to buy food would be to walk to a farm stand, buy what I needed for the next few days directly from the farmer, then walk home again. Yet for a city dweller like myself, that seemed more like a dream than a reality—until a few years ago, when a farmers' market opened in my neighborhood. In fact, this open-air gathering, where many local farmers sell their fruits and vegetables directly to shoppers, is even better than going to a roadside stand. In my town and in many others, the farmers' market not only carries a vast variety of produce, it's a great place to run into friends and neighbors, people-watch, and even hear music and see cooking demonstrations. Many farmers' markets are like one big street fair.

In most cases, you really can't beat the fruits and vegetables. I love to walk down the aisles and see stacks of rosemary, basil, and other fresh herbs on one table, corn piled high on the next. You can find an absolutely perfect nectarine at some farmers' markets and, at others, tomatoes that range in color from green to golden yellow to the more traditional red.

The reason that the produce at farmers' markets seems especially wonderful is that it's so up-to-the-minute fresh. The majority of the markets have rules stipulating that only producers who farm within a certain radius of the market can be vendors. That means that the produce you buy came from just a few miles away and was probably left on the vine until it achieved peak flavor, then was picked that morning or the night before. By contrast, the produce you buy at most supermarkets is usually picked before it reaches peak flavor so that it doesn't rot during transit, which can sometimes take days. That's why the produce (and particularly the fruit) you buy at a farmers' market usually tastes better than the prematurely picked produce you get in a supermarket. It's often more nutritious, too, since fruits and vegetables lose nutrients as they sit around in trucks and on store shelves.

When you buy produce from a farmers' market, you are also helping to support family farms and maintain rural areas close to where you live. Although the prices really aren't much higher at farmers' markets than at regular supermarkets (some fruits and vegetables are more costly, some are cheaper, so they balance out), farmers make more money selling directly to you than to grocery stores because they don't have to pay a middleman.

I personally try to buy as much organic produce as possible, which is another reason I'm a fan of farmers' markets. Not all vendors at farmers' markets sell organic food, but many of them do, and those who don't often use very few pesticides. Farmers' markets are also great places to get introduced to fruits and vegetables you've never tried before and to get some instruction on what to do with various kinds of produce. If you ask a grower how to use an herb such as lemongrass, a vegetable such as kohlrabi, or a fruit such as gooseberries, chances are you'll get a few interesting ideas. Some farmers even hand out recipes.

As of this writing, there are close to 3,000 farmers' markets around the country and the number keeps growing. So if you don't have one near you yet, don't give up hope; one may be on its way. I've visited markets in many different cities, and I've found that they vary quite a bit from one another. Some markets, for instance, allow vendors to sell vegetables and fruit only, while others permit baked goods and other prepared foods.

I find that prepared foods, such as hummus made from a farmer's own chickpeas or whole-grain breads, can be another terrific thing to buy at a farmers' market. One caveat: unlike commercially prepared foods, which are required to carry nutrition labels, farmers' market wares don't have to give you the specifics (calorie count, fat content, and so on). That leaves you a bit in the dark about what you're getting. On the bright side, you have someone on the other side of the booth to ask what went into the product—and I suggest you do just that before buying.

Natural Food Supermarkets

Just a few years back, the only stores that sold whole grains, soy products, and organic produce were the cramped little markets known as health food stores, and their selections were usually pretty limited. I don't want to knock them because for years they were the only stores offering health-conscious shoppers many options; however, in many cities and suburbs we now also have other choices: natural food supermarkets such as Whole Foods, Wild Oats, Fresh Fields, and Trader Joe's, to name just a few. There's been an explosion of these markets, which sell everything the little health food stores do, only more of it and in a much more stylish setting. They also carry organically fed beef and poultry, often have excellent seafood counters, and have aisles and aisles of nutritious convenience foods.

Some of these supermarkets are chains, with stores all over the country. What I appreciate about them is that they acknowledge that people who like to eat healthfully also care about how their food tastes. There is a world beyond brown rice and steamed vegetables, and these stores make it available to us by offering gourmet olive oils and mustards next to bins of whole grains such as bulgur; tasty fruit ices down the aisle from free-range eggs and organic milk; low-sugar, preservative-free cereals around the corner from jars of pure almond butter. If you like wholesome food, these markets are like heaven on earth.

Walking into one can be a bit of a rude awakening when it comes to money. Eating healthfully can be expensive, especially if you buy some of the more gourmet items. I have found that one of the best ways to take advantage of these great markets, but also keep costs down, is to go there for specialty items—such as organic meats, whole-wheat pasta, dried porcini mushrooms, and flavored vinegars—that are hard to find in supermarkets. Then I go to the regular market for paper goods and staples such as spices and canned tuna. It's a little more time-consuming—especially when you throw in a weekly trip to the farmers' market for produce—but I find that it's worth it.

Health Food Stores

If one of the big chain natural food markets hasn't come to your area yet, your best bet may be a small health food store. Many people have the idea that these stores carry only offbeat items such as gluten cakes and amino acid food additives, but in fact they are great places to buy things such as canned beans, nutritious soups, and organic tomato sauces. Small health food stores often carry good low-fat cheeses, whole-grain crackers, fresh smoothies, creamy nonfat and low-fat yogurts, and a wide assortment of nuts and nut butters. You can also generally find organic produce at these smaller stores, and they're a great place to buy things such as lentils and rice in bulk.

Regular Supermarkets and Grocery Stores

Maybe it's the fact that we're becoming a more nutrition-conscious country, maybe it's the competition from the natural food supermarkets, but whatever the reason, lots of supermarkets are starting to carry some healthier foods. Many even have special sections devoted to a wide variety of natural foods and carry organic produce, free-range poultry, and grass-fed beef. So even if the market near you doesn't specialize in natural or health foods, don't assume that it doesn't offer any. You just have to scrutinize the shelves; chances are you'll find something worthwhile.

Next time, for instance, before you toss the same old not-particularly-healthy cereal into your basket, stop and check out what else is there. Take some time to read the labels on cereals you've always passed by. There may be something there that you've been missing.

It's also a good idea to see if your market has a section of international and ethnic foods. Sometimes markets have just a few feet devoted to these foods, but there you may find a few interesting food choices such as black beans, salsas, basmati rice, miso soup, buckwheat soba noodles, and condiments such as curry paste that spice up food without adding many calories.

When you don't find items that you'd like to buy, try asking. Introduce yourself to the store manager, and see if he or she would be willing to order some of the items in which you're interested. At the very least, make your voice heard so that the manager knows there's an interest in healthy foods in your community.

Internet Shopping

For a while there, it seemed as though buying groceries over the Internet was the wave of the future. With the dot-com bust, that doesn't seem to be the case, but, you can still use your browser to good effect. Most food companies have Web sites, and on many sites you can order food to be delivered. You can even order organic produce, poultry, and meat. At the very least, you can usually log on to a manufacturer's Web site in order to find out where in your area you can buy its products. When I discover a product I like, I'll often go to the company's Web site to see what else it makes. Sometimes a manufacturer makes a whole range of great products but your store carries only part of its line. Checking out its Web site will clue you in to other foods you might like to seek out and try.

Tips for Making Healthful Choices

You know the basics when it comes to making healthful choices, but I want to help you further by putting different kinds of foods, and even specific products, onto your radar screen. These shopping tips will help you find foods that are not just nutritious but taste delicious—and that's key. Ultimately, you're not going to eat the healthy foods you buy unless they're appealing. To make eating well a lifelong habit, you have to get satisfaction, not just nutrients, from food.

Finding Great Fruits and Vegetables

- **Venturing outside the box.** Some of the problems people have with getting enough fruits and vegetables into their diet have to do with the boredom factor—they limit themselves to a very small range of options (fruit is an apple or orange, vegetables are iceberg lettuce and tomatoes). I urge you to branch out by trying things you don't usually buy. Tired of carrots and celery for snacks? Why not keep sliced bell peppers on hand instead? Spinach is not the only green that makes a good side dish. You may find that the earthier flavors of kale and Swiss chard appeal to you. Have you ever tried kiwi or papaya for breakfast instead of half a cantaloupe? For the most part, fruits and vegetables bought in season are relatively inexpensive, so experimenting won't be too costly.

- **Getting the most intense flavors.** If you've ever bought a peach in the middle of winter only to be greatly disappointed by how flavorless it was, you'll understand the value of eating seasonally. That peach was probably grown somewhere in the Southern Hemisphere, where it was summer, then shipped north. The trouble is, in order for the peach to withstand all that travel time, it has to be picked before it ripens properly (fruits soften after they're picked, but they don't get sweeter—that happens only on the vine). That means you're going to get a piece of fruit that tastes lousy.

  Eating seasonally—that is, consuming what the farmers in your area are harvesting that time of year—will ensure that you get produce that tastes as wonderful as it should. Besides, there is something wonderful about waiting all year for something such as tomatoes to come into season, then finally seeing the first batch at the farmers' market or grocery store. The anticipation makes everything taste that much better.

- **Take advantage of "convenience" foods.** You have no doubt noticed that many grocery stores now carry bags of precut and prewashed fruits and vegetables. (Even farmers' markets now carry some prewashed and premixed salad greens.) When I first saw them, I thought that buying them was a little too extravagant—you do, after all, have to pay more for the convenience—but then I began to realize that it really pays off in the end. If you buy fresh produce only to let it go bad in the crisper because you don't feel like triple-washing the spinach to get out all the sand or chopping up zucchini to put on top of your pasta, your money is going to waste anyway. Some of the bagged veggies may even inspire you to try new fruits and vegetables. I've seen bags of three kinds of Swiss chard (red, green, and yellow) and mixes of collard and beet greens. Emptying a bag into a pan with a little olive oil and garlic or into a pot of soup is a great way to get more of these superhealthy greens into your diet.

Exploring Whole Grains

- **Try a new cereal.** If you don't usually eat whole-grain cereals, one of the easiest ways to introduce yourself to them is to eat oatmeal. A lot of people, in fact, don't even know that oatmeal is a whole grain or that there are different kinds of oatmeal. Two of my favorites are McCann's Irish Oatmeal and Quaker Old-Fashioned Rolled Oats. Nutty and chewy, McCann's Irish Oatmeal is made with oats that are minimally processed. If you like a smoother texture, Quaker Old-Fashioned Oats, are rolled so they're not as chewy. Both companies make other kinds of oatmeals with various cooking times. Irish oatmeal takes more than half an hour to cook, so it's a good choice when you have some time. Regular old-fashioned oats take about five to ten minutes. If you're in a rush, there are quick-cooking and instant oatmeal, which you can even microwave. If you do buy instant oatmeal, choose the unflavored packets and sweeten the oatmeal yourself with a few drops of maple syrup since flavored instant oatmeal typically contains a lot of sugar. Granola is another oat-based cereal that contains a lot of flavor and is wonderful, but store-bought kinds can be packed with fat and sugar. Look for low-fat and low-sugar varieties (they *are* out there!) or try the granola recipe on page 108 instead.

  Commercial ready-to-eat cereals often contain preservatives (not to mention a lot of sugar—even the whole-grain ones) so I prefer the natural brands. They're not that hard to find these days; even some supermarkets carry them. When you buy a cereal, look at the ingredients list and make sure that it contains whole grains. Whole-wheat flour is a whole grain. Wheat flour is not.

- **The best breads.** Many people who were confirmed white bread eaters have made the switch to whole-grain bread, at least for toast and sandwiches. There are so many variations on the theme now— seven-grain bread, sprouted wheat bread, flaxseed bread—and manufacturers have refined their baking techniques to make these loaves very enticing. What's sometimes harder to give up is white French and Italian breads, those crusty loaves that go so well with soups and salads and lift sandwiches out of the ordinary. But whole-grain versions of these breads are out there (though unfortunately hardly ever served in restaurants), and I think you may come to like them if you buy good ones. Instead of trying the loaves you find in stores, introduce yourself to crusty-whole-grain breads by going to a bakery and buying loaves that have come out of the oven just hours before. Bakery loaves tend to be fresher and tastier. When you do buy store-bought sandwich loaves, follow the same rules you do when you buy cereals. Make sure the first ingredients on the list are whole-grain flours.

- **Better than white rice.** Maybe you've tried whole grains such as bulgur wheat or quinoa or whole wheat couscous—and decided never to try them again. Most of us have had a lifetime of eating white rice and regular pasta, so it's not surprising that it takes time to acquire a taste for these less refined variations. But I hope you won't give up on them yet. When you eat whole grains in dishes (anything from grain salads to side dishes and soups) that are well spiced, they are much more acceptable to the palate.

   Some of the recipes in this book may help you—Polenta with Swiss Chard and Portabella Mushrooms, for instance (many people don't realize that polenta is a whole grain). There are also some great grain mixes on the market that are worth trying. Near East Foods and Fantastic Foods make things such as tabouleh mix (a Mideastern dish made with bulgur wheat) that are both convenient and tasty. If you want to try various whole grains on your own, I suggest going to a market or health food store with bins of grains, which make it easy to buy small samples (no use getting stuck with a pound of quinoa, a light, but chewy grain, if you find you don't like it). Sometimes the bins will have cooking instructions; I copy them down and put the directions in a jar with the grain so I remember how to cook them.

Whole-wheat pasta is one of the whole-grain foods that people find particularly hard to switch to. Some whole-wheat pastas are less "grainy" than others. I recommend trying different brands until you find one you like.

Buying Meat, Poultry, and Fish

- **At the meat counter.** The kinds of meats, poultry, and fish you buy will depend on what your local stores carry and how much you are willing to spend. It's a given that you should select lean cuts of meat and poultry, but I also recommend that you seek out organic animal foods whenever possible. When an animal food is labeled "organic," it means that the livestock or poultry it comes from receives organic feed and is not given antibiotics and other medications. What an animal eats matters, because when you eat it, any antibiotics, hormones, or medications it has been fed may end up in your system, too. If you care about the treatment of animals (which I do), food from free-range animals is a good choice, too. "Free-range" means that the animal is not kept in a pen but rather is allowed to roam and eat grass. Unfortunately, free-range and organic meats and poultry are more expensive. They may fit into your budget or they may not, but if they do, I hope you will consider buying these healthier cuts of meat and poultry as often as you can.

- **Fish.** If you buy the freshest fish possible, it's going to taste better and you're going to be more likely to enjoy it. Frozen fish doesn't taste as good as fresh; however, frozen shrimp can be perfectly delicious. They're great to have on hand to throw into pasta or to cook in curry sauce and serve over brown rice. Another convenient form of seafood is tuna in the can and, now, in resealable packets. This is a recent innovation that makes it easy to tote tuna along to work (spoon it into your take-out salad). If you're reluctant to open a can because you hate the mess (and know you won't eat it all in one sitting), these resealable packets can make eating tuna even easier.

Dining Out—And Staying on the Program

So much of life these days revolves around eating in restaurants. Fast-food lunches. Too-tired-to-cook dinners. Business meals. Social get-togethers. Vacation dining. Special-occasion celebrations. Sometimes restaurant meals are just utilitarian: you eat out because it's convenient, because you're away from home, or because of professional demands. Sometimes it's about the food: you go to a place because it has a great chef. And sometimes it's just social: a restaurant meal is a pleasant way to spend time with friends or family. Unfortunately, all these meals, whether practical or pleasurable, can make it harder to lose weight and eat healthfully.

At home you have control over what goes into your meals. At restaurants, you can also have control, or at least a lot more control than you may think. I want you to seize that control so that you can enjoy dining out without undermining your commitment to the program. There's something relatively healthy on every restaurant menu—even those of restaurant chains such as Red Lobster, Sizzler, and Denny's, and fast-food eateries such as McDonald's and Wendy's.

I wouldn't recommend that you eat at fast-food restaurants often, but sometimes—as when you're on a three-hundred-mile road trip and there's nothing but fast-food places in sight—it can't be helped.

I'm happy to report, though, that fast-food menus are getting better all the time. You can now get salads (with fat-free or low-calorie dressings) at McDonald's, Wendy's, and Carl's Jr. Almost every fast-food place now also offers a grilled chicken sandwich (be sure to order it without mayonnaise or sauce), and Taco Bell has a soft chicken taco that is relatively healthy. Surprisingly, the simple single-patty hamburger is often the lowest-calorie sandwich on the menu at many fast-food restaurants (and also the lowest in saturated fat). It's when you order the double-patty cheeseburger that you get into trouble. Look for alternatives to sodas and milk shakes—many places now have low-fat milk, juice, and bottled water.

Most fast-food chains post menu nutrition information on their Web sites, so if you have Internet access, check it out before you go so you can plan ahead. Many fast-food restaurants also have the same information in a pamphlet or poster on the premises; ask for it before ordering.

It would be great if every restaurant had a pamphlet revealing the fat and calories in each dish it serves, but of course that's a rarity. Mostly you'll have to wing it, but I think you'll do fine if you follow these tips for dining out.

Before You Go Out the Door

- **Plan ahead.** I have a drawer that's devoted exclusively to menus from restaurants in my area. Leafing through the menus helps me think about what I'm really in the mood to eat so that I don't end up going someplace just because its convenient and end up having a meal that I didn't really want in the first place. My menu stash also lets me figure out what I'm going to order before I even get to the restaurant. That might sound unusual, but it really helps me stick to my resolve if I plan ahead.

  I recommend that you do the same. Collect menus from the restaurants you go to or are contemplating going to; many restaurants post their menus on their Web sites. In the clear light of your own home and without a server standing over you waiting to take your order, you can take the time to figure out what your best options are. Then, once you get to the restaurant, you'll be ready to order wisely.

- **Do your homework before you go on vacation.** Just as you plan where and what you're going to eat at home, prepare an eating strategy for when you're away. Look through guidebooks to find restaurants with healthy selections, and if you'll be staying at a hotel with a concierge, call ahead and ask him or her for suggestions. The concierge or restaurant you're interested in may even be able to fax you a menu at home.

- **Don't let yourself be pressured into dining out when you don't want to.** There are other places to have business meetings beside restaurants. Meet for tea or a drink, and order just a spritzer or some mineral water. There are other places to get together with friends besides a restaurant. Go to the movies and out for tea afterwards, not out to the movies and dinner. Consider entertaining at home so that you can make a healthy meal.

- **Eat a little something before you go out.** Have a small piece of fruit, some raw vegetables with a fat-free dip, or a whole-grain cracker with a little nut butter to take the edge off your hunger. There's nothing more dangerous than contemplating a menu full of dietary land mines when you're ravenous. You're likely to order much more than you really need.

Once You Get There

- **If possible, avoid getting steered to the bar.** Ever wonder why, when you show up for your reservation and the restaurant isn't full, they tell you that your table isn't ready and ask you to wait at the bar?

Restaurants make a lot of money from the sale of alcohol (even more money than they make from food), so they want to give you as much opportunity to drink as possible. But alcohol has a lot of hidden calories, and you should try to avoid it, or at least drink it in moderation. And remember, if you do end up in the bar, you're not obliged to order anything. If you must get something, order a juice spritzer (juice cut with carbonated water), which has half the sugar of juice, or just ask for a glass of water.

- **Decline wine and other alcoholic drinks.** As soon as you get to the table, your server will undoubtedly come around pushing more alcohol (a server always seems disappointed if you don't order a drink). Again, don't be pressured into ordering something that's not on your program. Lately, a lot of restaurants are also pushing bottled mineral water; yes, they overcharge, but it's healthy and you'll be much better off if you buy it instead of alcohol or soda. Just remember that carbonated water doesn't count toward your daily quota of eight eight-ounce glasses of water. However, many places also serve flat water, and that will count toward your quota.

- **Say no to the bread basket.** You think to yourself, "I'll just have one piece," but then you can't resist a second, and when your soup comes and you need something to mop up the last few drops from the bowl, you inevitably have a third. Suddenly you've eaten three pieces of bread, and your main course hasn't even come yet! After that much bread you'll probably feel pretty full, but you won't realize it and will end up eating your whole main course (instead of taking half of it home as you should if you're full). Make bread a nonissue. Decline the basket or ask your server to bring you one piece when your entrée comes.

- **Bond with your server.** To get what you want from the kitchen, you have to have a good relationship with your server. Make eye contact, explain what you want, ask questions. I frequently request to be in a particular server's section when I know he or she will be receptive to my requests. It's this person who'll be able to make sure that the vegetables I ordered are touched with olive oil, not soaked in butter, and that my fish is grilled, not pan-fried.

- **Don't be afraid to order off the menu.** The restaurant has everything you see on the menu—even if it's not always in the combinations you'd prefer. For instance, if a restaurant serves omelets, it has egg whites. If you prefer an egg-white omelet to the regular one on the menu, order it. If I see that the place I'm dining serves spaghetti with olive oil, I know it has olive oil—so I ask my server if they could grill a chicken breast with olive oil instead of serving it with a butter sauce. Want spinach in your pasta? If it's served as a side dish, they can toss it in with your noodles. When you read a menu, look at the ingredients, not just the dishes. Better restaurants will accommodate you—they want you to leave happy.

- **Split dishes with your dining partner or order creative combinations of appetizers.** The portions at most American restaurants are ridiculously large—and they keep getting bigger! So do yourself a favor: much as you may be against it on principle, pay the split charge (if the restaurant has one) and share a meal with someone at your table. Not only will you end up with a healthier meal, you'll actually save money since you won't have to pay for two entrées. Sometimes you don't even need to order an entrée at all; you can end up with a perfectly wonderful meal just by ordering a soup and an appetizer or two appetizers. Many finer restaurants will also shave entrées down to appetizer portions if you ask. Depending on with whom you're dining, you may get some flack for ordering lightly, but don't be swayed by what others want. Order the amount of food that's right for *you*.

After Dinner

- **If you wish, have a healthful dessert.** Opt for frozen yogurt, sorbet, or, best of all, fresh fruits. Instead of ordering from the dessert menu, you may even suggest that you and your dining companions go somewhere else. By the time you drive (or preferably walk) to the next place, you may realize that you're not even hungry for dessert anymore. When you order immediately after dinner, you haven't yet had the chance to get up and see how your body feels. The delay of going to another place will give you time to assess your appetite to see if you're really still hungry for dessert.

Being Good—But Not Perfect

I have a client who used to react badly to any kind of slipup. Whenever he would go off his program, even just slightly, he felt like such a failure that he would follow the slight slipup with a daylong eating spree. Then he would feel so bad about *that* that he would keep going, and it would take him *another* two to three days to get back on track. This man wasn't cutting himself any slack, a serious mistake; he was able to make headway only when he stopped beating himself up about going off the program and realized that it's human nature to occasionally eat things that aren't particularly healthy. In fact, he first experienced success when he began treating himself to something indulgent once in a while. He would enjoy it, realize that having a treat didn't mean that he was a terrible person with no willpower, and then resume eating healthfully.

One of the most important things you can do if you hope to reach your goals is to give yourself some freedom to occasionally eat unwisely. What's key, though, is that after it happens you then let it go. Move on. No one ever did a tremendous amount of damage to him- or herself at one meal, let alone in one day. But if you beat yourself up over a slipup, then one meal or one day of unhealthy eating can turn into days (or more) of destructive behavior and that will do damage.

I'm a firm believer in rewarding yourself for the hard work it takes to change lifelong behaviors, and sometimes this involves food. Maybe that means having an extravagant meal or a wonderful dessert now and again. My reward is an occasional lavish holiday meal or a delicious slice of pie. Because I don't have them very often, I don't take those holiday meals or that slice of pie for granted—I really enjoy them.

What helps, too, is that I make those indulgences a conscious act. I don't think of them as cheating, and neither should you. Think of them as something you deserve to have—which you do. Plan your treats, enjoy them, then get back onto the program. Don't let one indulgence set you off on a downward spiral of unhealthy eating.

It's also really important that you savor these rewards. There's nothing worse than feeding your emotions with just anything that's available. It should be a food that you really love or a favorite restaurant, not a food or place that's appealing simply because it's usually forbidden. You'll only be disappointed in the end and not feel the satisfaction you need to move on. Remember, too, that treats don't have to be unhealthy to be satisfying. One of my purposes in providing the dessert options in this book is to give you choices that are rewards for both your palate and, because they're nutritious, your body as well.

If after a small indulgence you wind up going off your program for days and can't seem to find it in you to get back on track, you need to dig deep to find out what's going on. What has caused you to backslide? This might be a time to turn to journal writing. Finding out what's behind your behavior is key to changing it.

That's one of the things that helped the client whom I described earlier get a handle on bingeing. Initially, when he first came to see me, he was bingeing seven days a week and not exercising. He started exercising regularly and got the bingeing down to five days a week, then three. Now it's only an occasional event because he learned what was behind the binges as well as to give himself rewards once in awhile. Of course, his goal is to stop the binges altogether, but he has already made dramatic progress by adding exercise to his life, putting his energy into understanding his destructive behavior, and choosing a healthy way of eating most of the time.

As you change your eating behavior, you're going to have good days and bad days. Concentrate on the good days. My guess is that you will spend more time eating well than eating poorly, so let that inspire you. Acknowledge your accomplishments, learn from your mistakes, and continue moving forward.

Although people vary in how much they struggle with over-indulging, the same is true for almost everybody: deprive yourself completely, and you are doomed to fail. Denial backfires. We all need rewards in life; just remember that food is only *one* way of rewarding yourself. It's so important to look at all the areas of your life and see how else you can reward yourself—or, if necessary, make changes. When food is your primary source of fulfillment you will always struggle with your weight. By the same token, if losing weight is your primary source of fulfillment, the numbers you read on the scale will forever dictate your mood. Examining your whole life and making an effort to improve each area that's important to you is the key to getting eating issues under control. Powerful change occurs over time by taking small steps toward all of your goals each day of your life.

PART III

Recipes

THE GOAL OF THE PRECEDING CHAPTERS was to help you get some new ideas about eating well. The goal of the following recipes is to help you put those ideas into practice. You know *how* to eat, now here's *what* to eat. My idea of a great recipe is one that combines sophisticated flavors with healthy ingredients, doesn't keep you in the kitchen for hours, and provides an enjoyable eating experience. The following recipes hit the mark in every way, as well as putting to rest the myth that nutritious eating is incompatible with pleasure. I think you'll find them nourishing for your body and spirit alike.

Most of the ingredients used to make these dishes are readily available and will probably be familiar to you. But if you haven't tried some of them, I hope these recipes will inspire you to branch out and try something new—in general, the more variety you can work into your diet, the healthier it will be. You may also be surprised to see that this recipe section includes some ingredients (cheese, sugar, and butter) and dishes (pastas, potato pancakes) that you don't normally find in a book devoted to nutritious eating. I believe that, in moderation and with some culinary ingenuity, you can work just about anything into your diet and still keep it healthful and nutritious.

Once you get cooking, I think you'll see exactly what I mean. Enjoy!

Breakfast

MOST DAYS, MOST PEOPLE have little time for breakfast. Some of the recipes in this section reflect that rush we all feel—they either take just a few minutes to make or can be prepared in advance so that you can eat them quickly and be on your way. Other recipes here require more time but are great for days when you have time for a more leisurely meal. Some of the egg dishes are great for lunch or dinner, too.

Peaches and "Cream" Fresh Fruit Smoothie

I like to have smoothies for breakfast because they provide great nutrition quickly and you can mix and match your favorite ingredients for a lot of variety. This smoothie is one of my favorites because it combines a rich, creamy texture with the taste of peaches.

SERVES 2

1 medium peach, peeled and seeded
½ medium banana
1 kiwifruit
½ cup low-fat or nonfat yogurt
½ cup orange juice
¾ cup ice cubes
Mint sprig, for garnish

In a blender or food processor, blend the peach, banana, kiwifruit, yogurt, and orange juice for about 1½ minutes or until the mixture is creamy and smooth. Add the ice and blend until creamy and smooth. Serve in a chilled glass with a sprig of mint.

Fresh Fruit Medley

Fruit gives you a burst of energy; that's why I love to include it in my morning meal. I can get tropical fruits easily, but feel free to substitute any of your favorite, locally available fresh fruits, for this dish. Have a serving of this for breakfast, and you've had your fruit for the day!

SERVES 2

½ medium kiwifruit, peeled and sliced on the diagonal

½ medium papaya, peeled, seeded, and sliced on the diagonal

½ medium mango, peeled, seeded, and sliced on the diagonal

½ medium banana, peeled and sliced on the diagonal

Mint sprigs, for garnish

½ cup plain low-fat or nonfat yogurt (optional)

¼ cup wheat germ (optional)

Arrange the sliced fruit on a chilled plate and garnish with mint sprigs. You can drizzle the fruit with yogurt and sprinkle with wheat germ; or place the yogurt and wheat germ in a small bowl and use it as a dip for the fruit, if desired.

Homemade Granola

Better than store-bought!

MAKES ABOUT 6 CUPS

3½ cups rolled oats

½ cup oat bran

½ cup whole raw almonds

½ cup apple juice concentrate

½ cup honey

1 teaspoon cinnamon

1 teaspoon pure vanilla extract

4 egg whites

¼ cup sugar

½ cup raisins or currants

Preheat oven to 350°F. Spread oats on a large nonstick baking pan and toast, stirring often, for 30 minutes. Cool. Reduce the oven heat to 275°F. In a large mixing bowl, combine the oats, oat bran, almonds, apple juice concentrate, honey, cinnamon, and vanilla. In a separate mixing bowl, whip the egg whites to soft peaks. Add the sugar and beat 1 minute more. Combine the oat mixture with the egg whites and spread evenly on a nonstick baking sheet. Toast for 30 minutes, stirring often, until evenly browned. When cool, add raisins or currants. Store in an airtight container.

Granola Yogurt Parfait

A delicious, satisfying breakfast—or dessert.

SERVES 4

2 cups granola

2 5-ounce containers nonfat flavored yogurt (such as vanilla
   or peach)

2 baskets ripe organic strawberries or any other fruit,
   washed and sliced

In four parfait or wine glasses, alternate layers of granola, yogurt, and strawberries to fill each glass ¾ full. Serve immediately.

Bran Muffins with Fruit

Make a batch and freeze some of these muffins. That way you'll always have a quick breakfast on hand.

MAKES 12 MUFFINS

2 cups bran

1 cup low-fat buttermilk

4 tablespoons canola oil

2 eggs

¼ cup brown sugar

¼ cup molasses

1 cup whole-wheat flour

1 teaspoon baking soda

¼ teaspoon salt

1 small carrot, grated

1 small apple, peeled and grated

½ small banana, mashed

½ cup currants

Preheat oven to 375°F. Spray a 12-cup nonstick muffin tin with cooking spray. In a large bowl, combine the bran, buttermilk, canola oil, eggs, sugar, and molasses. Set aside and let stand for 20 minutes to soften the bran. In a separate bowl, mix together the flour, baking soda, and salt. Add the flour mixture to the bran mixture. Stir in the grated carrot, apple, banana, and currants. Do not overmix. The batter should be lumpy. Fill the muffin cups halfway and bake for 15 to 20 minutes, or until a toothpick inserted into the center comes out clean.

Blueberry Buttermilk Pancakes

Adding blueberries to pancakes gives them a healthy shot of antioxidants (and a healthy shot of flavor, too).

12 5-INCH PANCAKES

SERVES 4 TO 6

¾ cup unbleached all-purpose flour

½ cup whole-wheat flour

1½ teaspoon baking powder

½ teaspoon salt

2 tablespoons sugar

¼ teaspoon baking soda

2 cups low-fat buttermilk

2 tablespoons canola oil

2 eggs, separated

Nonfat cooking spray

1½ cups blueberries, fresh or unthawed frozen

Maple syrup

Vanilla nonfat yogurt

Additional blueberries, for garnish

Sift the flours, baking powder, salt, sugar, and baking soda into a mixing bowl. In another bowl, beat together the buttermilk, canola oil, and egg yolks. Make a well in the flour mixture and pour in the buttermilk mixture. Stir lightly to incorporate. In a small clean and dry bowl, whisk the egg whites until stiff. Gently fold into the batter and let rest for 15 minutes. Spray a pancake griddle with nonfat cooking

continued

spray. Drop 2-ounce (¼ cup) portions of batter on the griddle and cook over medium-high heat. As the pancakes begin to set, sprinkle with a few blueberries. Continue to cook until the batter is bubbly and the bottom is brown, about 2 minutes. Turn and cook 1 minute more. Repeat until the batter is used up. Serve at once with maple syrup, yogurt, and more blueberries.

Potato Pancakes

These make a delicious weekend breakfast, a light lunch, or even a
Sunday-night supper.

SERVES 2

1 egg, separated
1 large baking potato, peeled, coarsely grated, and
    thoroughly drained
1 medium onion, finely chopped
1 teaspoon finely chopped chives
Pinch of baking powder
2 teaspoons flour
Salt and pepper to taste
Nonfat cooking spray
Plain low-fat or nonfat yogurt
Unsweetened applesauce

Heat a nonstick skillet over a medium flame. In a bowl, beat the egg
white until it holds stiff peaks. In a large bowl, mix together the potato, onion, chives, baking powder, flour, and egg yolk. Fold in the egg
white and salt and pepper. Spray the skillet with cooking spray. Drop
the batter by tablespoonfuls onto the skillet. Brown well on one side,
then flip and brown on the other side. Serve immediately with yogurt
and applesauce on the side.

Scrambled Egg Whites with Spinach and Orange

With the added flavor of tomato, cayenne and orange, you won't miss the yolks.

SERVES 2

6 egg whites

2 tablespoons tomato sauce

Nonfat cooking spray

4 ounces fresh spinach, well washed and stems trimmed

Dash of cayenne pepper

Salt to taste

Grated rind of one orange

Beat the egg whites until frothy, then blend in the tomato sauce. Heat a skillet over a medium flame and spray with cooking spray. Sauté the spinach until it is wilted and there is no liquid in the pan. Pour in the egg whites, season with cayenne pepper, and salt and cook slowly, stirring until thickened. Sprinkle with grated orange rind and serve immediately.

Potato Omelet

This omelet is baked, not cooked on top of the stove.

SERVES 2

Nonfat cooking spray
1 medium onion, finely chopped
1 cup mashed potatoes
3 eggs, separated
3 tablespoons soy milk
1 tablespoon finely chopped parsley
Salt and pepper
Sliced tomatoes

Preheat the oven to 350°F. Spray an ovenproof skillet with cooking spray. Over medium heat, sauté the onions. Place the potatoes in a bowl, add the egg yolks and soy milk, and beat until smooth. Stir in the onions and chopped parsley. Season to taste with salt and pepper. Beat the egg whites until stiff and fold gently into the potato mixture. Wipe out the skillet and spray with cooking spray. Pour in the batter and bake for about 20 minutes, until the top of the omelet is brown; fold over and turn onto a platter. Serve with sliced tomatoes.

Poached Eggs with Veggie Hash

Precooking the potatoes makes this breakfast a quick project. Precook the potatoes the night before or use leftover diced roasted red potatoes.

SERVES 4

VEGGIE HASH

3 medium-size russet potatoes, peeled and diced

2 tablespoons olive or canola oil

1 medium onion, diced

1 red bell pepper, seeded and diced

1 yellow bell pepper, seeded and diced

1 tablespoon chopped parsley

½ teaspoon paprika

Salt and freshly ground pepper

POACHED EGGS

8 cups cold water

½ teaspoon salt

2 tablespoons white vinegar

8 fresh eggs

Bring 1 quart salted water to a boil. Drop in the diced potatoes and cook until al dente, slightly undercooked. Handle carefully, or you will have mashed potatoes! Drain the potatoes in a colander and cool with running cold water. Dry well, or the potatoes will not become crispy and brown.

Pour 1 tablespoon oil into a nonstick pan over medium-high heat. Add the potatoes and cook to golden brown, stirring occasionally.

When brown, push the potatoes to one side, add the onion and 1 tablespoon oil, stir in the peppers, and cook until lightly browned. Stir together in the pan. Sprinkle with parsley, paprika, salt, and pepper. Divide among four bowls and top with 2 poached eggs each.

The vinegar ensures that the egg whites will set. Eggs that are not fresh will not produce a well-formed poached egg.

Bring the water to a boil in a shallow pan. Add the salt and vinegar. Reduce to a slow simmer. Break 2 eggs into a small bowl, then slide into the simmering water. Repeat with all the eggs. Cook until set. Two minutes produces a soft poach. Remove from the water with a slotted spoon.

Breakfast Fried Rice (With or Without the Rice)

Two thirds of the world's population begin their day with a bowl of rice. And so can you!

This is a quick stir-fry, so you want to have all of your ingredients chopped and ready. To make this a really quick dish, microwave the leftover rice and keep it hot. If you omit the rice, you will have a tasty scrambled egg dish with Asian flavors.

SERVES 4

2 tablespoons canola oil

½ cup sliced mushrooms

½ cup celery, thinly sliced diagonally

4 scallions, sliced diagonally

½ cup snow peas, ends stripped off and cut in half
   diagonally

½ cup bean sprouts

6 eggs, beaten

1 cup leftover cooked rice, reheated

Dash of light soy sauce

Salt and freshly ground pepper

In a large nonstick pan heat 1 tablespoon canola oil over medium-high heat. Starting with the mushrooms, stir-fry the vegetables, adding the celery, scallions, snow peas, and bean sprouts in sequence. Remove the vegetables from the skillet. Add the eggs and scramble them lightly. Add 1 tablespoon canola oil and the hot cooked rice. Stir to combine. Add the cooked vegetables to the rice and egg mixture. Season with a dash of soy sauce, salt, and pepper.

Soups

SOUPS ARE A SECRET WEAPON in the fight against extra pounds. Many soups—including the ones here—are low in calories but extremely filling. I recommend starting a meal with a serving of soup. It's so satisfying, you'll be likely to eat less if you do. Or make a meal of soup. Served with some crusty whole-grain bread, each of these recipes is great on its own as lunch or a light supper.

Roasted Tomato Soup

A deeply flavored tomato soup accented with herbs.

SERVES 4

3 pounds Roma tomatoes, washed and cored

1 medium onion, chopped

1 tablespoon minced garlic

1 tablespoon olive oil

A few sprigs of fresh thyme or oregano

1 cup low-fat, low-sodium chicken stock

1 12-ounce can evaporated skim milk or 12 ounces
   1 percent milk

Salt and freshly ground pepper

Toasted croutons, for garnish

Chopped fresh herbs, such as basil, parsley, or chives,
   for garnish

Preheat the oven to 350°F. Place the tomato, onion, and garlic on a nonstick baking sheet or a baking sheet that has been sprayed with nonfat cooking spray. Drizzle with olive oil. Tear up the fresh herbs and sprinkle them over the tomatoes, onion, and garlic. Bake for 30 minutes, until the tomato skins are lightly charred and broken. Place the tomatoes, onion, and garlic in a soup pot and add the chicken stock. Bring to a simmer and cook for 15 minutes. Puree the soup in batches in a food processor, then strain through a large-holed sieve, pressing down on the solids with a ladle to extract all of the juices and pulp. Discard the skins, seeds, and herb stems. Return the soup to the pot, heat to a simmer, and add the milk. Season to taste with salt and pepper. Ladle into warmed bowls and garnish with croutons and chopped fresh herbs.

Red Tomato Gazpacho

This soup takes a little bit of effort, but it's worth it. The hand-chopped vegetables give the soup a delightful crunch.

SERVES 4

6 large vine-ripened tomatoes, peeled, seeded, and chopped

2 cucumbers, peeled, seeded, and diced

1 red pepper, seeded and diced

1 green pepper, seeded and diced

1 small red onion, diced

2 cloves garlic, minced

1 bunch of fresh basil, leaves cut into thin strips

1 bunch of cilantro, leaves chopped

1 small serrano chile, minced

1 46-ounce can low-salt tomato juice

1 cup red wine vinegar

¼ cup extra-virgin olive oil

Water, if necessary

Salt and freshly ground pepper

In a large bowl, combine the tomatoes, cucumbers, peppers, onion, garlic, basil, cilantro, chile, tomato juice, vinegar, and olive oil. Stir, cover, and chile for at least 6 hours, and preferably overnight. When ready to serve, thin to the desired consistency with cold water and season to taste with salt and pepper.

Mushroom Soup

For a more complex flavor, this soup is best made with two or three kinds of mushrooms. A few rehydrated dried mushrooms (such as dried porcini) added to the broth give it an even meatier flavor.

SERVES 4

1 pound mixed mushrooms, such as button, shiitake, oyster, portabella, and crimini

A few dried porcini mushrooms, rehydrated (optional)

2 tablespoons olive oil

1 large onion, chopped

1 teaspoon minced garlic

⅓ cup sherry (optional)

1 quart low-fat, low-sodium chicken stock or vegetable stock

1 russet potato, peeled and diced

1 tablespoon chopped fresh thyme or 1 teaspoon dried thyme

1 bay leaf

1 12-ounce can evaporated skim milk

Salt and freshly ground pepper

Clean and chop the mushrooms, including the dried porcini, if using. Discard the shiitake mushroom stems. Heat the olive oil in a soup pot over medium heat. Add the onion and garlic and cook, stirring occasionally, until opaque but not brown. Add the mushrooms and continue cooking with a lid on until the mushrooms are cooked, about 10 minutes. Add the sherry, if desired, bring to a boil to cook off the alcohol, then add the chicken stock, potato, thyme, and bay leaf. Simmer until the potato is tender. Remove bay leaf and puree in batches in a food processor or blender. Return to the pot and add the evaporated skim milk. Bring just to a boil and season to taste with salt and pepper.

Gingered Butternut Squash Soup

Perfect for a crisp fall day. Use fresh nutmeg if you can—it really makes a difference.

SERVES 4

1 tablespoon olive oil

1 small onion, diced

1 butternut squash, peeled and diced

1 knob of fresh ginger, about 1 inch long, peeled and finely chopped

1 small carrot, peeled and chopped

6 cups low-fat, low-salt chicken stock

1 bay leaf

¾ cup 1 percent milk or evaporated skim milk

Salt and freshly ground pepper

¼ teaspoon nutmeg, or to taste, freshly ground if possible

Chopped chives or scallions, for garnish

In a soup pot over medium-high heat, place the olive oil and onion. Cook, stirring often, until the onions are softened. Add the squash, ginger, carrot, chicken stock, and bay leaf. Cover and simmer until all the vegetables are soft, about ½ hour. Puree the soup in batches in the blender. Thin the soup with the milk and season to taste with salt, pepper, and nutmeg. Garnish with chopped chives or scallions.

Leek and Potato Soup

I like to use Yukon Gold potatoes in this hearty, creamy soup, but russets will do just fine.

SERVES 4

1 tablespoon olive oil

1 small onion, peeled and chopped

1 large leek, quartered lengthwise, well washed, and chopped

2 large potatoes, peeled and chopped

4 cups low-fat, low-salt chicken stock

1 bay leaf

1 12-ounce can evaporated skim milk or 12 ounces 1 percent milk

Salt and freshly ground pepper

In a soup pot over medium-high heat, heat the olive oil. Add the onion and leek and cook, stirring, until the vegetables are softened but not brown, about 5 minutes. Add the potatoes, chicken stock, and bay leaf and bring to a boil. Reduce the heat and simmer, covered, for about 30 minutes, or until the potatoes are very tender. Add the milk and remove from the heat. Puree the soup in batches in a blender or food processor. Return to the pot and, if necessary, thin with a little more milk or stock. Season with salt and pepper and serve hot in heated bowls.

Corn Chowder

Chiles give this hearty soup a southwestern flavor.

SERVES 4

1 tablespoon olive oil

1 medium onion, diced

1 celery stalk, diced

1 teaspoon minced garlic

2 cups corn kernels, cut from the cob

1 large russet potato, peeled and diced

2 teaspoons ground cumin

1 teaspoon chili powder

Pinch of cayenne pepper

1 bay leaf

4 cups low-fat, low-salt chicken stock

2 pasilla chiles, roasted, peeled, seeded, and diced, or one
    small can Ortega roasted chiles

1 red bell pepper, roasted, peeled, seeded, and chopped, or
    one small jar roasted red peppers

2 tablespoons cornstarch

1 12-ounce can evaporated skim milk or 12 ounces
    1 percent milk

Salt and freshly ground black pepper

1 large bunch cilantro, leaves coarsely chopped, for garnish

In a soup pot, heat the olive oil over medium-high heat. Add the
onion, celery, and garlic and cook until softened, stirring often, about
5 minutes. Add the corn, potato, cumin, chili powder, cayenne pep-

per, bay leaf, and chicken stock. Bring to a boil, reduce the heat, and simmer for 30 minutes. Add the roasted chiles and red bell pepper. Stir the cornstarch into the milk and stir the mixture into the soup until the soup thickens slightly. Do not allow to boil. Season with salt and pepper. Ladle into warmed bowls and garnish with chopped cilantro.

Provençal Vegetable Soup (*Soupe au Pistou*)

This classic summer soup from the South of France is filling enough to serve as a light supper. You may have some *pistou* left over; try it tossed with some whole-wheat spaghetti.

SERVES 4

1 tablespoon olive oil

1 medium onion, finely chopped,

1 small leek, white part only, well washed and finely chopped

1 large carrot, peeled and chopped

2 stalks celery, chopped

1 small zucchini, diced

1 cup green beans, cut into 1-inch lengths

8 cups low-fat, low-salt chicken stock

½ cup cooked or canned, drained navy beans

1 large potato, peeled and diced

1 14-ounce can diced tomatoes

2 ounces fine pasta, such as vermicelli, broken into small pieces

Salt and freshly ground black pepper

PISTOU

3 cloves garlic, peeled

Leaves from 1 large bunch basil

Juice of one lemon

4 tablespoons freshly grated Parmesan cheese

Cooking liquid from the soup

4 tablespoons extra-virgin olive oil

Salt and freshly ground black pepper

Over medium heat, heat the olive oil in a large soup pot. Add the onion, leek, carrot, celery, zucchini, and green beans. Cook, stirring, until the vegetables are softened, about 5 to 10 minutes. Add the stock and the navy beans. Bring to a boil and reduce the heat. Simmer, covered, for about 15 minutes. Add the potatoes, tomatoes, and pasta and cook, covered, another 10 to 15 minutes, until the potatoes and pasta are cooked through. Season with salt and pepper.

MAKE THE *PISTOU:*

In the bowl of a food processor, combine the garlic, basil, lemon juice, Parmesan and 2 tablespoons of the cooking liquid from the soup. Process for about one minute. Slowly add the olive oil until all are well combined; season with salt and pepper.

Ladle the soup into bowls and spoon a little of the *pistou* into each serving.

Curried Lentil Soup with Yogurt

A spicy treat. You may add more curry powder or cayenne pepper to increase the heat, or even a chopped chili. The yogurt is a cooling contrast to the spicy soup.

SERVES 4

1 tablespoon olive oil

1 small onion, chopped

1 medium carrot, peeled and chopped

2 stalks celery, chopped

1 garlic clove, minced

1 tablespoon curry powder

Pinch cayenne pepper

1 bay leaf

1 cup dried lentils, washed and picked over

3 cups low-fat, low-salt chicken stock or water

Salt and freshly ground pepper

¼ cup plain nonfat yogurt

Thinly sliced scallions, for garnish

In a soup pot over medium-high heat, heat the olive oil. Add the onions, carrot, celery, and garlic. Cook until softened but not brown, about 5 to 10 minutes, stirring often. Add the curry powder and cook another 2 minutes to release the flavor of the spices. Add the cayenne pepper, bay leaf, lentils, and stock or water. Bring to a boil, reduce the heat, and cover. Simmer for about 45 minutes, checking occasionally to make sure there is enough liquid in the pot; you may need to add more stock or water. Season with salt and pepper. Ladle into warmed bowls and garnish with yogurt and scallions.

Red Bean Soup

A warming soup for a cool evening.

SERVES 2

5 ounces dry red kidney beans, soaked overnight

Nonfat cooking spray

2 slices turkey bacon, chopped

1 medium onion, chopped

1 garlic clove, peeled and crushed

1 medium carrot, peeled and chopped

1 stalk celery, chopped

1 bay leaf

1 sprig thyme or ½ teaspoon dried thyme

1 teaspoon sugar

1 teaspoon cayenne pepper

1 teaspoon ground cumin

Salt and freshly ground pepper

Cooked rice, for garnish

Drain the beans and rinse well under cold running water. Spray a soup pot with cooking spray and over medium heat sauté the bacon, onion, and garlic for about 5 minutes. Add the carrot and celery and cook 2 minutes more. Pour in the water and bring to a boil. Add the beans, bay leaf, and thyme and reduce the heat. Cover and simmer about 30 minutes, or until the beans are tender. Remove the bay leaf and thyme and add the sugar, cayenne pepper, cumin, salt, and pepper. Stir to combine and cook about 5 minutes more. Puree the soup in batches in a blender or food processor until smooth. Return soup to the pot and reheat; taste and adjust the seasonings. Serve sprinkled with cooked rice.

Fish Chowder

This tasty soup makes a delicious summer supper. Be sure to wear gloves when working with the Scotch bonnet pepper, and don't touch your eyes or lips until after you've washed your hands.

SERVES 2

8 ounces snapper fillets, cut into strips

Juice of one lemon

2 tablespoons chopped cilantro leaves

Salt and freshly ground pepper

Nonfat cooking spray

1 leek, top and bottom trimmed, split lengthwise, and cut into 1-inch slices, well washed

1 garlic clove, minced

½ Scotch bonnet pepper, seeded and minced

6 large vine-ripened tomatoes, skinned, seeded, and cut into chunks, juice reserved

1 large potato, peeled and cut into 1-inch chunks

1 cup clam juice

In a nonreactive bowl, toss the fish with the lemon juice, cilantro, salt, and pepper. Cover and refrigerate until ready to use, but no more than ½ hour. Spray a 2-quart pot with cooking spray, and over medium heat sauté the leek until soft, about 5 to 10 minutes. Add the garlic and Scotch bonnet pepper. Add the tomato, reserved juice, potato, and clam juice and simmer about 15 minutes. Stir in the snapper and any liquid in the bowl. Simmer for 10 minutes; taste and adjust the seasoning. Serve immediately.

Salads, Small Plates, and Sandwiches

SOMETIMES YOU DON'T WANT a big meal. When you're in the mood for something light—at lunch, at dinner when you've had a big mid-day meal, or when you're simply not very hungry—try the recipes in this chapter. A couple of the dishes from this chapter may be all you need to feel satisfied.

Salads have come a long way since the days of tossed iceberg and vinaigrette, and the ones in this chapter are no exception. Many of them combine greens or other vegetables with wonderful little extras such as toasted walnuts and small amounts of cheese. Some of them work as accompaniments to a meal; others are meals in themselves. Try them in combination with a bowl of soup, a sandwich, or one of the small plates.

The possibilities are endless!

Fruity Green Salad

This simple salad combines different flavors and textures to tantalize your taste buds.

SERVES 2

2 ounces arugula leaves, well washed and dried, end and middle stems removed

½ cucumber, peeled, seeded, and cut into thin strips

½ bulb fennel, sliced as thinly as possible

1 ripe Bartlett pear, peeled, cored, and thinly sliced, lengthwise

1 tablespoon chopped flat-leaf parsley

Juice of one lemon

4 tablespoons light olive oil

Salt and freshly ground pepper

1 ounce Parmesan cheese, thinly shaved

In a large bowl, combine the arugula, cucumber, fennel, pear slices, and parsley. In a small bowl, combine the lemon juice, olive oil, salt, and pepper. Whisk together, pour over the salad, and toss well. Serve at once, garnished with the shaved Parmesan.

Baby Greens with Warm Goat Cheese and Walnut Vinaigrette

This is a sophisticated salad that could begin an elegant dinner or make a delicious light lunch. You can find walnut oil at a well-stocked supermarket, gourmet store, or health food store.

SERVES 4

WARM GOAT CHEESE

4 teaspoons finely chopped walnuts

1 tablespoon fresh bread crumbs

1 teaspoon chopped chives

1 teaspoon chopped parsley

1 4-ounce log of fresh goat cheese, cut into 4 rounds

WALNUT VINAIGRETTE

3 tablespoons walnut oil

3 tablespoons olive oil

2 tablespoons red wine vinegar

1 shallot, minced

Salt and freshly ground pepper

4 cups baby greens or mesclun mix, washed and dried

8 cherry tomatoes, cut in half

Slices of French bread, toasted, for garnish (optional)

continued

Preheat the oven to 350°F. Combine the walnuts, bread crumbs, chives, and parsley in a small bowl. Press the mixture onto all sides of the goat cheese rounds. Place the rounds on a nonstick baking sheet and bake for 5 to 8 minutes, until warmed through.

Whisk together all the ingredients for the vinaigrette and toss with the greens. Divide among four plates. Top each plate with a goat cheese round and 4 tomato halves, and serve with toasted French bread, if desired.

Crispy Romaine Salad with Apples, Celery, Toasted Walnuts, and Light Blue Cheese Dressing

This salad is full of the flavors of autumn.

SERVES 4

LIGHT BLUE CHEESE DRESSING

6 tablespoons extra-virgin olive oil

2 tablespoons red wine vinegar

1 shallot, minced

2 tablespoons blue cheese crumbles

Salt and freshly ground black pepper

4 hearts of romaine lettuce, washed, dried, and left whole

1 Granny Smith apple, cored and thinly sliced

2 stalks celery, cut into thin diagonal slices

2 tablespoons toasted walnuts

Freshly ground black pepper

MAKE THE LIGHT BLUE CHEESE DRESSING:

In a small bowl, whisk together all the ingredients until well combined. Set aside.

Divide the romaine hearts among four chilled plates. Divide the apple, celery, and walnuts evenly over the lettuce. Drizzle 1 tablespoon of the dressing over each plate. Grind pepper over each plate and serve immediately.

Asparagus Vinaigrette

The quintessential spring salad.

SERVES 4

1 pound asparagus

VINAIGRETTE

2 tablespoons red wine vinegar

1 shallot, minced

Kosher salt and freshly ground pepper

6 tablespoons extra-virgin olive oil

2 hard-cooked eggs, finely chopped

1 small red onion, finely chopped

1 tablespoon chopped parsley

Freshly ground pepper

Break off the tough ends of the asparagus stalks; the stalks should be about the same length. Either steam or boil the asparagus until tender but still bright green. Plunge the cooked stalks into a bowl of ice water. Drain and dry the stalks, and divide among four plates.

MAKE THE VINAIGRETTE:

In a small bowl, whisk together the vinegar, shallot, salt, and pepper. Gradually add the olive oil, whisking, until the dressing is emulsified.

Drizzle the vinaigrette over the asparagus. Scatter the eggs, onion, and parsley evenly over the plates. Serve and pass the additional pepper.

Fresh Summer Tomato Salad with Fresh Mozzarella and Basil

This salad should be made only with vine-ripened tomatoes. I like to use red, golden, and cherry tomatoes from my local farmers' market.

SERVES 4

VINAIGRETTE

6 tablespoons extra-virgin olive oil

2 tablespoons red wine vinegar

½ teaspoon minced garlic

Salt and freshly ground pepper

2 pounds assorted vine-ripened tomatoes

1 ball (4 ounces) fresh mozzarella

Leaves from 1 bunch fresh basil, cut into thin slices, some
   whole leaves reserved for garnish

Salt and freshly ground black pepper

In a small bowl, whisk together the olive oil, vinegar, garlic, salt, and pepper. Set aside. Core the larger tomatoes and cut into wedges; cut cherry tomatoes in half. Slice the mozzarella in half lengthwise and cut each half across into four pieces. Place the tomatoes, mozzarella, and basil in a bowl. Whisk the vinaigrette and pour over the salad. Toss gently, and let sit at room temperature for 15 minutes. Divide the salad among four plates and garnish with whole basil leaves. Season with salt and pepper.

Summer Tomato Salad

This salad takes a little effort, but it's well worth it.

SERVES 4

VINAIGRETTE

2 tablespoons balsamic vinegar

1 tablespoon Dijon mustard

6 tablespoons extra-virgin olive oil

Salt and freshly ground pepper

2 pounds assorted vine-ripened tomatoes

Leaves from 1 bunch of basil, thinly sliced

1 small red onion, thinly sliced

2 teaspoons drained capers

2 tablespoons Niçoise or Kalamata olives, pitted

1 cup ½-inch homemade croutons*

In a small bowl, combine the vinegar and mustard. Slowly whisk in the olive oil and season with salt and pepper. Set aside.

Core the larger tomatoes and cut into wedges; cut cherry tomatoes in half. Place them in a large bowl and add the basil, onion, capers, olives, and croutons. Drizzle with the vinaigrette and toss gently. Let stand for at least 15 minutes. Divide among four plates and serve.

---

* To make croutons: Slice French or Italian bread ½ inch thick; cut each slice into cubes. Place the cubes in a bowl and drizzle with olive oil. Toss. Place the cubes on a baking sheet and toast in a 350°F oven for approximately 15 minutes, or until crisp.

Green Bean Salad with Toasted Walnuts

I like to use slightly bitter lettuces in this dish. If you can't find frisée, arugula or endive is a good substitute. Roasted beets are a delicious addition to this salad.

SERVES 4

1 pound green beans, ends removed

1 head frisée lettuce, washed and torn into bite-sized bits

1 small red onion, thinly sliced

VINAIGRETTE

2 tablespoons red wine vinegar

1 shallot, minced

1 teaspoon chopped fresh thyme

Salt and freshly ground pepper

6 tablespoons extra-virgin olive oil

4 tablespoons toasted walnuts

4 teaspoons crumbled blue cheese

Steam or boil the green beans until tender-crisp, about 5 minutes. Plunge the beans into ice water, drain, and dry well. In a large bowl, place the beans, frisée, and onion.

MAKE THE VINAIGRETTE:

In a small bowl, whisk together the vinegar, shallot, thyme, salt, and pepper. Slowly whisk in the olive oil.

Pour the vinaigrette over the salad and toss gently. Divide the salad among four plates, and garnish each with a tablespoon of walnuts and a teaspoon of blue cheese.

Wild Rice Salad

The nutty flavor and chewy texture of wild rice, accented with fruits and nuts, makes this a satisfying starter, an elegant accompaniment, or a light entrée.

If you can't find Belgian endive, substitute butter lettuce.

SERVES 4

¾ cup wild rice

½ teaspoon salt

½ cup pecan halves

4 tablespoons currants or dried cranberries

CITRUS VINAIGRETTE

2 tablespoons lemon juice

1 tablespoon sherry vinegar

6 tablespoons olive oil

1 tablespoon minced shallot

Grated zest of one small orange

Salt and freshly ground pepper

2 heads Belgian endive

½ cup diced celery

1 green apple, cored, peeled, and diced

1 tablespoon chopped parsley

Cover the rice with water and soak for about ½ hour. Drain the rice. Bring 1 quart of water to a boil. Add the salt and rice. Reduce the heat to a simmer, cover, and cook about 35 to 40 minutes, until the rice grains are open and tender. When the wild rice is cooked, drain in a colander and allow to cool to room temperature. Preheat the oven to 350°F. Place the pecan halves on a baking sheet and toast for 10 to 15 minutes. Remove from the oven and set aside. Place the currants or cranberries in a heatproof bowl and cover with boiling water for 5 to 10 minutes. Drain and set aside.

MAKE THE CITRUS VINAIGRETTE:

Place the lemon juice and vinegar in a small bowl. Slowly whisk in the olive oil to emulsify. Add the shallot, orange zest, and salt and pepper to taste and whisk to combine.

ASSEMBLE THE SALAD:

Cut off the root ends of the endives and separate the large outer leaves. Lay the leaves in a bicycle spoke pattern around a serving plate. Chop the inner endive leaves into 1-inch pieces and put them into a small bowl. Add the rice, celery, currants or cranberries, pecans, and apple. Toss with the Citrus Vinaigrette and correct seasoning. Mound the rice mixture in the middle of the endive spokes. Sprinkle the plate with chopped parsley.

Tuna with Grape Tomatoes and Greens

This is a salad for people on the go: filling, high in protein, and rich in fiber.

SERVES 2

8 stalks asparagus, cooked and cut into 2-inch pieces

1 6-ounce can albacore white tuna in water, drained

6 ounces cooked chickpeas, drained

6 leaves romaine lettuce, washed, dried, and shredded

½ cucumber, peeled, seeded, and cubed

12 grape tomatoes, halved

1 tablespoon capers

1 tablespoon chopped cilantro

Juice of ½ lemon

1 tablespoon white wine vinegar

1 teaspoon soy sauce

1 teaspoon Tabasco

4 tablespoons peanut oil

Salt and freshly ground black pepper

In a salad bowl, place the asparagus, tuna, chickpeas, lettuce, cucumber, and tomatoes. In a small bowl, whisk together the capers, cilantro, lemon juice, vinegar, soy sauce, Tabasco, peanut oil, and salt and pepper to taste. Drizzle the dressing over the salad and toss gently to coat all the ingredients. Serve immediately.

Salade Niçoise

The traditional Salade Niçoise is a beautiful summer entrée. A composed salad, it always includes cold potatoes, green beans, ripe tomatoes, olives, capers, hard-cooked eggs, and an anchovy or two. If you use a light hand with the salty ingredients, this can be a healthful treat. Most recipes call for tuna, but in this variation I use a 3-ounce portion of grilled or poached salmon, and I leave out the anchovies.

SERVES 4

1 pound green beans, cooked until tender-crisp

2 medium beets, roasted and cut into wedges

1 pound small red potatoes, roasted and halved

2 large vine-ripened tomatoes, cored and cut into wedges

4 3-ounce salmon fillets, grilled or poached

4 hard-cooked eggs, peeled and halved

2 teaspoons capers

6 Niçoise olives

VINAIGRETTE

2 tablespoons red wine vinegar or lemon juice

1 shallot, minced

Salt and freshly ground pepper

6 tablespoons extra-virgin olive oil

1 tablespoon chopped parsley or basil

continued

On four plates, arrange the green beans, beets, potatoes, and tomatoes in a bicycle wheel spoke pattern. Place a piece of salmon in the center of each plate. Garnish with a hard-cooked egg half. Sprinkle with the capers and olives.

MAKE THE VINAIGRETTE:

Whisk together the vinegar or lemon juice, shallot, salt, and pepper. Slowly add the olive oil, whisking until well combined.

Drizzle 1 tablespoon of the dressing over each salad and sprinkle with the chopped parsley or basil.

Marinated Italian Seafood Salad

The flavors of the Mediterranean on a plate. You may substitute flat-leaf parsley for the basil.

SERVES 4

½ pound medium shrimp, peeled and cleaned, tails left on

½ pound squid, cleaned, body cut into rounds, tentacles cut
    in half if they are large

2 stalks celery, thinly sliced

1 small red pepper, thinly sliced

1 small red onion, thinly sliced

8 Kalamata or Picholine olives, pitted and chopped

2 tablespoons drained capers

Leaves from 1 bunch of basil, thinly sliced

⅛ teaspoon hot pepper flakes, or to taste

2 tablespoons extra-virgin olive oil

1 tablespoon white wine vinegar

1 teaspoon minced garlic

Salt and freshly ground pepper

1 head butter lettuce, washed and separated into leaves

Lemon wedges, for garnish

Chopped parsley, for garnish

Bring a large pot of salted water to a boil. Add the shrimp and cook until they are pink and firm, about 1 minute. Remove from the water with a small sieve or slotted spoon and transfer to a bowl of ice water. Add the squid to the boiling water and cook for 30 to 45 seconds. Re-

continued

move with a sieve or slotted spoon and place in the ice water. Drain the cooked shrimp and squid well and place in a medium bowl. Add the celery, pepper, onion, olives, capers, basil, pepper flakes, olive oil, vinegar, garlic, salt, and pepper. Toss well and refrigerate, covered, for 2 hours.

Line four plates with lettuce leaves and divide the salad equally among the plates. Garnish with lemon wedges and chopped parsley.

Spicy Mexican Shrimp Cocktail

When it's too hot to think of cooking, this easy-to-make dish hits the spot.

SERVES 4

COCKTAIL SAUCE

1 small cucumber, peeled, seeded, and diced

2 Roma tomatoes, seeded and diced

¼ small yellow onion, diced

1 serrano chile, minced

2 tablespoons chopped fresh cilantro leaves

32 ounces Clamato juice

Juice of 2 limes

1 small avocado, diced

4 tablespoons ketchup

2 dashes Tabasco, or to taste

16 medium shrimp, peeled, cleaned, and cooked, or 2 cups
    defrosted bay shrimp

Lime wedges, for garnish

Baked Tortilla Chips (see below)

MAKE THE COCKTAIL SAUCE:

In a medium bowl, combine the cucumber, tomatoes, onion, chile, cilantro, Clamato juice, lime juice, avocado, and ketchup. Season to taste with the Tabasco. Let sit for 30 minutes.

Divide the sauce among four martini glasses. If using medium

continued

shrimp, hang four of them from the rim of each glass. If using bay shrimp, place ½ cup in each glass on top of the sauce. Garnish with lime wedges and serve with Baked Tortilla Chips.

Baked Tortilla Chips

4 corn tortillas
Nonfat cooking spray
Salt
Chili powder

Preheat the oven to 350°F. Cut each tortilla into six pieces and place on a nonstick baking sheet. Spray the pieces with cooking spray and season with the salt and chili powder. Bake until the chips are crisp, 10 to 15 minutes. Turn the baking sheet twice to ensure that the chips cook evenly. Allow to cool slightly before serving.

Hummus with Toasted Pita Triangles

Pair this with the Roasted Tomato Soup (page 120) for a light lunch.

MAKES ABOUT 2½ CUPS

2 cups cooked chickpeas, drained

1 tablespoon olive oil

2 teaspoons minced garlic

1 tablespoon tahini

2 tablespoons lemon juice (1 lemon yields about
    1 tablespoon of juice)

Warm water

Salt and freshly ground pepper

2 scallions, sliced, for garnish

1 teaspoon toasted sesame seeds, for garnish

Toasted Pita Triangles (see below)

Assorted raw vegetables (carrot and celery sticks, cucumber
    slices, bell pepper slices)

In a food processor, puree the chickpeas, olive oil, garlic, tahini, and lemon juice. Thin the puree with warm water until it is the consistency of a dip; season with salt and pepper.

Mound the puree in a bowl, garnish with the sliced scallions, and sprinkle with sesame seeds. Serve with Toasted Pita Triangles and raw vegetables for dipping.

continued

Toasted Pita Triangles

4 pita breads
Nonfat cooking spray
Salt

Preheat the oven to 400°F. Cut each pita into eight pieces. Place the pieces on a nonstick baking sheet. Spray the pieces with the cooking spray and sprinkle lightly with salt. Bake until crisp, about 10 minutes. Cool slightly before serving.

Tomatoes Stuffed with Couscous, Cucumber, and Mint

This light entrée is actually a snap to make, and looks so impressive!

SERVES 4

4 large vine-ripened tomatoes

Salt and freshly ground pepper

1 cup couscous

1 cup boiling water

1 small cucumber, peeled, seeded, and diced

1 tablespoon fresh mint leaves, thinly sliced

1 tablespoon chopped fresh parsley

1 tablespoon extra-virgin olive oil

Juice of one lemon

1 tablespoon pine nuts

2 scallions, both white and green parts, minced

2 cups baby lettuce or mesclun mix

Cut off the tops of the tomatoes and hollow them out. Season with salt and pepper and turn them upside down on a paper towel to drain.

Place the couscous in a heatproof bowl and pour the boiling water over. Cover tightly and let it sit for 20 minutes. Uncover and fluff the couscous with a fork, making sure there are no lumps.

Cool the couscous to room temperature and add the cucumber, mint, parsley, olive oil, lemon juice, pine nuts, and scallions. Season with salt and pepper. Mound the couscous into the tomatoes and serve on a bed of greens, lightly dressed with olive oil and a squeeze of lemon juice.

Eggplant and Zucchini Poor Boy Sandwich

One very satisfying vegetarian sandwich, coming right up!

SERVES 4

1 small eggplant

1 medium zucchini

1 medium red onion

Nonfat cooking spray

4 tablespoons olive oil

Salt and freshly ground pepper

2 tablespoons finely chopped Kalamata or green olives

1 tablespoon chopped fresh oregano

1 teaspoon finely chopped garlic

2 tablespoons feta cheese

1 large vine-ripened tomato, thinly sliced

1 long loaf crusty Italian bread or four rolls

Cut off the ends of the eggplant and slice into ½-inch rounds. Trim the zucchini and cut lengthwise into ¼-inch slices. Cut the onion into ¼-inch slices. Lay the cut vegetables on a nonstick baking sheet that has been sprayed with cooking spray. Brush the vegetables with olive oil and season with salt and pepper; let them sit at room temperature for 30 minutes. Preheat the oven to 450°F and bake the vegetables for 10 to 15 minutes, turning once. (You could also grill the vegetables.)

Combine the olives, oregano, and garlic with the feta cheese. Slice the bread or rolls in half and toast lightly. Layer the eggplant, zucchini, and onion on one half and sprinkle with the feta mixture. Top with the sliced tomato. Close the loaf or rolls; if using a loaf, slice it into four portions.

"Grilled" Veggie Burgers

When you're craving a hamburger, try this instead. There are a number of delicious vegetable burgers available in your grocer's frozen food case. Just pick your favorite one for this recipe.

SERVES 2

Nonfat cooking spray

1 small onion, halved and thinly sliced

1 portabella mushroom cap, thinly sliced

1 small red pepper, seeded, halved, and thinly sliced

1 tablespoon soy sauce

2 veggie burgers

4 slices whole grain bread

2 slices low-fat Swiss cheese

Spray a skillet with cooking spray. Sauté the onion for 1 minute; add the mushroom and pepper and cook, stirring, until the vegetables are soft, about 5 to 10 minutes. Add the soy sauce and stir. Remove the vegetables from the skillet to a plate.

Spray both sides of the veggie burgers with cooking spray and cook, about 3 to 4 minutes per side or according to the package instructions. Toast the bread. Place each burger on a slice of bread and top with a slice of cheese and the sautéed vegetables. Cover with the remaining slices of bread, cut in half, and serve immediately.

Portabella Mushroom Burgers

Here's another vegetarian answer to that burger craving. It's a little work, but the end result is a gourmet's delight. If you don't want to grill the mushrooms, which have a great meaty flavor, they can be roasted in a 350°F oven in a foil-covered baking dish for about 30 minutes. Serve these with dill pickle spears and Healthy Coleslaw (page 188).

SERVES 4

4 large portabella mushroom caps
2 tablespoons olive oil
Salt and freshly ground pepper
½ teaspoon chopped fresh thyme
2 garlic cloves, sliced

2 large red onions, cut into ½-inch rings
1 tablespoon olive oil

4 ounces soft fresh goat cheese
½ teaspoon chopped fresh thyme
1 clove garlic, minced

4 whole-grain burger buns, lightly toasted
1 or 2 large vine-ripened tomatoes
½ small head romaine lettuce, thinly sliced

Rub the mushrooms with the olive oil, salt, pepper, thyme, and garlic. Marinate at room temperature for 15 minutes.

Preheat the oven to 350°F. Toss the onion rings with 1 tablespoon olive oil, salt, and pepper. Place on a nonstick cookie sheet and roast in the oven for 15 to 20 minutes. Stir occasionally to cook evenly or until cooked through. Remove from the oven and keep warm.

In a bowl, mix the goat cheese with salt, pepper, thyme, and minced garlic. Set aside.

Grill or roast the mushrooms. Slice them diagonally, and lay one mushroom on the bottom of each of the toasted buns. Divide the onions over the mushrooms. Spread the other half of each bun with some of the goat cheese mixture. Top the mushrooms with sliced tomatoes and lettuce. Cut each sandwich in half.

Salmon Burger

The secret to this sandwich is that the fish must be absolutely fresh.

SERVES 2

12 ounces salmon fillet, skin removed

1 shallot, chopped

2 egg whites

¼ red pepper, finely chopped

¼ green pepper, finely chopped

Salt and freshly ground black pepper

2 tablespoons fresh bread crumbs

Nonfat cooking spray

2 kaiser rolls, sliced in half

2 teaspoons Dijon mustard

4 arugula leaves, well washed and dried

2 slices ripe tomato

1 teaspoon chopped fresh dill

On a clean chopping board with a very sharp knife, dice the salmon very fine. Place in a medium-sized bowl with the shallot. In a small bowl, whisk the egg whites until frothy. Combine with the fish, shallots, diced pepper, and salt and pepper to taste. Gently fold in the bread crumbs and form into two patties. Heat a skillet over medium-high heat. Spray both sides of the patties with cooking spray and cook 3 to 4 minutes on each side. Toast the rolls and spread the mustard on both sides. On the bottom half of the roll, mound the arugula and tomatoes and place the cooked burger on top. Sprinkle with dill, close the roll, and enjoy.

Artichoke and Tuna Panini

Panini are small Italian sandwiches made with rustic Italian rolls flavored with rosemary, olives, or a salt glaze. They're terrific served with a simple green salad.

SERVES 4

4 large crusty rolls

2 6-ounce cans albacore tuna packed in water

8 to 10 baby artichokes, packed in water

4 tablespoons chopped roasted red peppers, store-bought or homemade

4 teaspoons chopped olives, such as Niçoise or Kalamata

4 tablespoons thinly sliced basil leaves

4 teaspoons olive oil

Fresh ground pepper

Juice of one lemon

Cut the rolls in half and remove some of the bread to form a pocket. Set aside. Drain the tuna. Cut the artichokes into quarters lengthwise. On the bottom half of each roll, layer the tuna, artichokes, peppers, olives, and basil. Drizzle with the olive oil and season with the pepper. Sprinkle with the lemon juice. Replace the top half of the roll and press down on the panini. Cut in half to serve.

Entrées

DINNER IS THE MEAL MANY PEOPLE LOOK FORWARD to the most. It shouldn't disappoint, and none of these entrées does. Each is exceptionally flavorful, but also light, so that you don't leave the table feeling weighed down—a feeling you want to avoid as your body (and your metabolism) is winding down for the day. You may notice that I haven't included any red meat among these recipes. That's because most people get more than their fair share of beef and other red meats, and I'd like to encourage you to limit your intake. Whether you decide to give up red meat completely is a personal choice, but at the very least, eat it in moderation. And here are some good substitutes. Chicken, turkey, seafood, vegetarian dishes—I think you'll find these main dishes entirely satisfying.

Tofu and Broccoli Stir-Fry

The secret of a good stir-fry is to have all of your ingredients at hand, sliced, chopped, minced, and measured before you begin, so that you can proceed quickly. That way the end result will be vegetables that are crisp and colorful, not soggy or discolored by overcooking. Start with the longest-cooking item first and continue adding, finishing with the bean sprouts and green scallions. Do not add all of the oil at once but as it is needed, a tablespoon at a time.

If you can find baby bok choy, use it here.

Serve the stir-fry with steamed brown rice.

SERVES 4

1 tablespoon canola oil

½ cup sliced shiitake mushrooms, stems discarded,
   or ½ cup sliced button mushrooms

1 tablespoon sesame oil

1 cup broccoli crowns, stems sliced thinly and florets cut
   into small pieces

1 cup bok choy, cut into 2-inch pieces

1 teaspoon minced garlic

1 tablespoon grated fresh ginger root

1 pound firm tofu, drained and cut into 1-inch cubes

1 cup low-fat, low-salt chicken or vegetable stock

1 cup bean sprouts

2 tablespoons light soy sauce

2 tablespoons sliced scallions

2 tablespoons chopped fresh cilantro

Salt and freshly ground pepper

Heat a wok or large heavy skillet over high heat until hot. Add 1 tablespoon oil and stir-fry the mushrooms. Add the sesame oil, broccoli, bok choy, garlic, and ginger. Stir-fry until the vegetables just begin to soften. Add the tofu and vegetable or chicken stock. Cover and heat through, about 1 minute. Finally, add the bean sprouts and stir well to heat through. Stir in the soy sauce, scallions, and cilantro. Season to taste with salt and pepper.

Vegetable Frittata

Serve this light entrée with a simple salad of baby greens. The frittata can be served hot or at room temperature.

SERVES 4

6 eggs

1 tablespoon chopped parsley

Salt and freshly ground pepper

2 tablespoons olive oil

1 small onion, diced

1 cup sliced mushrooms

½ pound cooked asparagus tips

1 large red potato, cooked and cut into ¼-inch slices

1 Roma tomato sliced ¼-inch thick

4 teaspoons grated Parmesan cheese

Preheat the oven to 350°F. In a small bowl, beat the eggs with parsley, salt, and pepper; set aside. Heat a medium-size ovenproof nonstick skillet. Add 1 tablespoon olive oil and cook the onion until lightly browned, about 7 to 10 minutes. Add the mushrooms and cook, stirring often, until the mushrooms are cooked through and all the liquid has evaporated. Remove the onions and mushrooms from the pan and set aside. Wipe the pan clean, return to the heat, and add the remaining olive oil to the pan. Over medium-high heat, add the eggs and cook for 3 to 4 minutes, until they begin to set. Sprinkle the onions, mushrooms, asparagus, potatoes, and tomato over the top. Sprinkle with the Parmesan cheese and put the skillet in the oven for about 5 to 10 minutes, until the cheese melts. Slide the frittata onto a serving dish and cut into quarters.

Spinach Penne with Spicy Roasted Pepper Sauce

Use whole-wheat pasta. Jerk seasoning can be found in the spice section of your grocery store.

SERVES 2

3 red bell peppers, cut in half lengthwise, seeded, and ribs
    removed
2 teaspoons jerk seasoning
8 ounces penne
Salt
4 tablespoons olive oil
1 onion, halved and thinly sliced
10 ounces fresh spinach, well washed and stems removed
1 tablespoon thinly sliced basil leaves
Grated Parmesan cheese or crumbled fresh goat cheese

Preheat the oven to 350°F. Rub the inside of the peppers with the jerk seasoning. Lay them cut side down on a baking sheet and roast for 45 minutes or until the skin is black. Put the peppers in a bowl and cover with plastic wrap until cool. Cook the penne in salted boiling water for about 8 minutes. Drain and toss with 2 tablespoons of olive oil. Rub the skins off the cooled peppers. Place the flesh in a food processor with the juices from the bowl and baking sheet and process until smooth.

In a large skillet over medium-high heat, sauté the onions in the remaining olive oil for about 2 minutes. Add the spinach and cook until the onions are soft and the spinach is wilted. Pour the penne and the pepper mixture into the pan and cook over medium heat until the penne is completely coated with sauce. Divide between two plates and sprinkle with the basil and cheese.

Broccoli and Swiss Chard Cannelloni

A classic reinvented with a nutritious addition of broccoli and chard.

SERVES 4

FILLING

2 cups low-fat ricotta cheese

2 tablespoons grated Parmesan cheese

½ cup steamed broccoli, chopped

½ cup steamed Swiss chard, drained and chopped

½ cup sautéed chopped onion

1 tablespoon minced garlic

½ teaspoon nutmeg

1 egg

Salt and freshly ground pepper

PASTA

4 sheets fresh pasta or 4 sheets frozen, thawed pasta sheets

Nonfat cooking spray

TOPPING

1 28-ounce can marinara sauce or 2 cups homemade marinara sauce (recipe below)

Parmesan cheese, to taste

In a large bowl, thoroughly combine all the filling ingredients. Cut the pasta sheets into 4-by-5-inch rectangles. Cook briefly in boiling salted water, a few at a time, then drop them into a bowl of ice water. Remove from the ice water and lay out on a damp kitchen towel.

Spray the pasta squares with nonfat cooking spray, which will prevent them from sticking to one another.

Spray a rectangular nonstick baking pan with nonfat cooking spray and set aside. Preheat oven to 400°F. Divide the filling among the eight rectangles of cooked pasta, rolling them up and placing them seam side down on the baking pan. Top with the marinara sauce, sprinkle with a little grated Parmesan cheese, and bake until the sauce is bubbling and the cannelloni is heated through, about 15 minutes.

Marinara Sauce

2 tablespoons olive oil
1 large onion, chopped
2 stalks celery, chopped
1 tablespoon minced garlic
½ cup white wine
1 28-ounce can crushed tomatoes plus 1 19-ounce can
   crushed tomatoes
1 bay leaf
Leaves from 1 bunch of fresh basil, thinly sliced
Pinch of sugar
Salt and freshly ground pepper
Pinch of chili flakes (optional)

Heat a saucepan over medium-high heat. Add the olive oil, onion, celery, and garlic. Cook, stirring often, until translucent but not browned. Add the white wine and bring to a boil. Add the crushed tomatoes, bay leaf, and basil. Reduce the heat to a simmer, cover, and cook for 20 minutes. Season with a pinch of sugar, salt, pepper, and optional chili flakes. Simmer a few more minutes to blend the flavors.

Polenta with Swiss Chard and Portabella Mushrooms

Polenta provides a nice change of pace from pasta and it's creamy texture makes it a great (albeit healthy) comfort food.

SERVES 4

2 tablespoons olive oil

¼ cup chopped onion

1 teaspoon minced garlic

2 large portabella mushroom caps, thinly sliced

1 large bunch Swiss chard, well washed, large stems removed, and leaves torn into bite-size pieces

Salt and freshly ground pepper

2 cups low-fat, low-salt chicken stock

½ cup polenta

¼ cup grated Parmesan or Asiago cheese

Chopped parsley, for garnish (optional)

Heat a large nonstick pan over medium-high heat. Add 1 tablespoon of olive oil to the pan and sauté the onion and garlic until soft, about 5 minutes. Add the remaining olive oil and add the mushrooms. Cook until soft, about 3 to 5 minutes. Add the Swiss chard and 2 tablespoons of water to the pan. Cover and cook until the chard is wilted, about 4 minutes. Season the mixture with salt and pepper and set aside.

In a 2-quart saucepan, bring the chicken stock to a boil. Gradually add the polenta, whisking constantly. When all the polenta is added, lower the heat to medium and continue to cook, stirring often, for about 20 minutes. Season with salt, pepper, and the grated cheese. Divide the polenta among four serving dishes and top with the reserved mushroom-chard mixture. Sprinkle with chopped parsley, if desired.

Steamed Manila Clams and Mussels in White Wine Broth with Chili Flakes and Spaghetti

Manila clams are small, tender farm-raised clams about the size of a small mussel. Littleneck clams may be substituted if you cannot find Manila clams, but they take longer to cook.

Serve with a big green salad.

SERVES 4

2 pounds Manila clams

2 pounds mussels

1 pound spaghetti

3 tablespoons extra-virgin olive oil

Salt and freshly ground black pepper

½ cup minced shallots

1 tablespoon minced garlic

2 cups dry white wine

¼ cup chopped fresh parsley

Leaves from 1 bunch fresh basil, thinly sliced

½ teaspoon dried chile flakes, or to taste

Grated Parmesan cheese

Soak the clams and mussels in several changes of water for ½ hour. Scrub the clams and mussels with a brush and remove the beards from the mussels, if necessary. Discard any clam or mussel with a broken shell.

Cook the spaghetti in 4 quarts rapidly boiling water until al dente. Drain well, toss with one tablespoon of olive oil and salt, and keep warm.

Heat the remaining olive oil in a deep pot over medium-high heat.

Add the shallots and garlic and cook for about 3 minutes, stirring often. Add the wine, increase the heat to high, and let come to a boil. Add the clams and mussels, cover, and steam until they open, about 5 minutes. Add the chopped parsley, basil, and chile flakes. Divide the spaghetti among four bowls, then divide the clams and mussels on top of the spaghetti. Discard any unopened shells. Ladle the broth into each bowl carefully so you don't include any sand that might have been inside the clams or mussels. Sprinkle with a teaspoon of grated Parmesan cheese. Season to taste with freshly ground black pepper.

Pan-Seared Fillet of Tilapia with Mango Tomato Salsa and Lentil Pancake

Whoever thought that something this high in protein and fiber and low in fat could taste so good?

SERVES 2

2 6-ounce fillets of tilapia

Juice of one lemon

1 garlic clove, crushed

1 tablespoon chopped parsley

Salt and freshly ground pepper

MANGO SALSA

1 firm mango, peeled, flesh cut off the seed, and diced

1 tomato, peeled, seeded, and cut into ¼-inch dice

1 tablespoon chopped chives

4 tablespoons light olive oil

LENTIL PANCAKE

1 egg white

½ cup lentils, cooked until very tender and drained

¼ red bell pepper, seeded and diced fine

1 scallion, finely chopped

1 tablespoon flour

In a nonreactive bowl, place the fish, half the lemon juice, garlic, and parsley. Season with salt and pepper. Cover and refrigerate.

MAKE THE MANGO SALSA:

In a small bowl, combine the mango, tomato, chives, the rest of the lemon juice, and 2 tablespoons of olive oil. Season with salt and pepper and set aside for at least an hour.

MAKE THE LENTIL PANCAKES:

In a small bowl, whisk the egg white until fluffy. Fold in the drained lentils, red pepper, scallion, and flour. In a nonstick skillet over medium-high heat, make two even circles of the lentil mixture. Cook for about a minute on each side, then place each pancake on a serving plate.

Remove the fish from the marinade and pat dry. Spray both sides of the fillets with nonfat cooking spray. Sauté the fish about 5 minutes on each side, until golden brown. Lay a fillet over each pancake and garnish with the Mango Salsa.

Hoisin Shrimp and Okra with Brown Rice

The spicy sweetness of the shrimp is a pleasing contrast to the earthy flavor of the brown rice.

SERVES 2

8 ounces medium shrimp, peeled and deveined

Juice of one lemon

½ teaspoon grated ginger

4 ounces hoisin sauce

4 ounces brown rice

½ teaspoon salt

12 ounces chicken stock or water

2 tablespoons light olive oil

1 small onion, diced

1 garlic clove, minced

4 ounces okra, washed and cut into ½-inch-thick rounds

½ teaspoon fresh thyme

1 large ripe tomato, seeded and diced

Freshly ground pepper

1 scallion, finely chopped

In a nonreactive bowl, place the shrimp with half the lemon juice, the ginger, and the hoisin sauce. Cover and refrigerate for about an hour.

Put the rice, salt, and stock or water in a heavy pan. Bring to a boil, reduce the heat, and cook, covered for about 45 minutes.

In a medium skillet, heat the olive oil over medium-high heat. Sauté the onion and garlic until soft, about five minutes. Very gently stir in the okra and the thyme, stirring as little as possible so the okra doesn't become "slimy." Add the rest of the lemon juice, the tomatoes, and salt and pepper to taste and cook an additional 5 minutes. Add the marinated shrimp and the scallions, mix gently, and cook 5 minutes more. Serve the shrimp and okra over the rice.

Baked Lemon Herb Halibut

I serve this with brown rice or steamed baby red potatoes.

A good rule for cooking fish is to allow 10 minutes of cooking time for each inch of thickness. Professional chefs always pull fish from the oven when it is slightly underdone, as it will continue to cook while you plate and serve it.

SERVES 4

Nonfat cooking spray
4 5-ounce skinless halibut fillets
Salt and freshly ground pepper
⅓ cup chopped scallions
3 tablespoons chopped fresh dill
3 tablespoons chopped fresh tarragon
3 tablespoons chopped fresh parsley
4 tablespoons extra-virgin olive oil
1 cup dry white wine or vermouth (optional)
One lemon, sliced very thinly, for garnish

Preheat the oven to 350°F. Spray a shallow baking pan with cooking spray. Place the fillets in the pan and season with salt and pepper. Cover the fillets with the scallions, dill, tarragon, and parsley, drizzle with olive oil, and pour the wine or vermouth, if desired, around the fish. Bake for 10 to 15 minutes. Baste the fish with the pan juices once or twice and serve some of the juices with each fillet. Garnish with lemon slices.

Mustard-Crusted Baked Salmon

This dish is relatively simple, but the flavors are complex—a real delight!

SERVES 4

4 5-ounce salmon fillets

Salt and freshly ground black pepper

Nonfat cooking spray

4 generous tablespoons whole-grain mustard

½ cup Quick Herbed Bread Crumbs (see below)

1 cup white wine or vermouth (optional)

2 tablespoons olive oil

Lemon wedges, for garnish

Preheat the oven to 350°F. Pat the fish dry and season with salt and pepper. Spray a shallow baking dish with cooking spray. Place the fillets in the dish. Coat the top of each fillet with one tablespoon of mustard, and press 1 generous tablespoon of Quick Herbed Bread Crumbs into the mustard to make a crust. Carefully pour the white wine or vermouth, if desired, around the fish and drizzle with the olive oil. Bake for 10 to 15 minutes, or until the fish is done. If the crust isn't sufficiently browned, you can briefly run the pan under the broiler.

Serve with the pan juices spooned around the fish and lots of lemon wedges.

continued

Quick Herbed Bread Crumbs

Remove the crusts from several slices of day-old French bread. Place the slices into a food processor and pulse until medium crumbs form. To ½ cup bread crumbs add 1 tablespoon each of chopped fresh thyme and parsley, 1 teaspoon minced garlic, and a drizzle of olive oil to bind the bread crumb mixture.

Grilled Tuna or Swordfish with Roasted Red Pepper Vinaigrette

I like to serve this with grilled asparagus.

SERVES 4

2 large sweet red bell peppers

2 tablespoons drained capers

2 tablespoons minced garlic

1 tablespoon chopped fresh thyme or leaves from one small
   bunch basil, sliced thin

1 tablespoon sherry vinegar

Salt and freshly ground pepper

4 5-ounce tuna or swordfish steaks

Nonfat cooking spray

Lemon wedges, for garnish

Preheat the broiler. Place the peppers on a foil-lined baking sheet and broil 2 inches below the flame, turning often, until blistered and charred on all sides. Transfer the peppers to a small bowl and cover with plastic wrap for about ½ hour. When the peppers are cool enough to handle, remove the skin, seeds, and stems. Cut the peppers into thin strips about 2 inches long and return to the bowl. Add the capers, garlic, thyme or basil, and sherry vinegar. Season with salt and pepper.

Prepare the grill or preheat the broiler. Season the fish with salt and pepper and spray each side with cooking spray. Cook the tuna about 2 minutes on each side; the swordfish should be cooked 3 to 5 minutes on each side, depending on its thickness.

Remove the fish from the grill, spoon the vinaigrette over, and serve garnished with lemon wedges.

Lemon Parsley Chicken Breast with Baby Artichokes and Potatoes

This one's for all lemon lovers!

SERVES 2

2 6-ounce skinless bone-in chicken breasts

2 shallots, peeled and quartered

Juice of two lemons

4 tablespoons chopped flat-leaf parsley

3 tablespoons light olive oil

Salt and freshly ground pepper

10 baby artichokes

2 baking potatoes, peeled and cut into ¼-inch-thick strips

In a nonreactive dish, place the chicken breast with the shallots, juice of one lemon, 3 tablespoons parsley, 1 tablespoon olive oil, salt, and pepper. Turn to coat, cover, and refrigerate. Prepare the artichokes by cutting off the stem even with the base. Snap off about three layers of outer leaves, slice off about an inch of the tops, and cut in half lengthwise. Place in a bowl of water with the juice of half a lemon.

Preheat oven to 400°F. Remove the chicken from the marinade and place in a shallow baking pan. In the bowl in which the chicken was marinating, place the remaining lemon juice and olive oil and season with additional salt and pepper. Remove the artichokes from the water and pat dry; toss them and the potatoes in the olive oil–lemon mixture. Arrange the vegetables around the chicken and bake for about 25 to 30 minutes. After the first 15 minutes, gently turn the vegetables. Remove the chicken and vegetables to a platter and serve sprinkled with the remaining parsley.

Grilled Skinless Chicken Breasts with Mango-Tomato Salsa

Serve this with warm corn tortillas and Black Beans (page 199).

If you cannot find fresh mango, you can use fresh pineapple or papaya. Flattening the chicken breasts is optional, but you'll find they cook more evenly if they're a uniform thickness.

SERVES 4

1 ripe mango, peeled, pitted, and diced

2 large tomatoes, peeled, seeded, and diced

1 serrano chile, minced (more if you like spicy food)

1 tablespoon minced red onion

1 small bunch cilantro, leaves chopped

Juice of one lime or lemon

A few dried chile flakes

1 scallion, minced

2 tablespoons olive oil

Salt and pepper

4 5-ounce boneless, skinless chicken breasts

In a bowl, place the mango, tomatoes, chile, onion, cilantro, lime or lemon juice, chile flakes, scallion, olive oil, and salt and pepper. Mix well and let sit for 30 minutes to let the flavors blend.

Place the chicken breasts between two sheets of plastic wrap and flatten with a rolling pin to a uniform thickness. Over a medium-hot charcoal grill, using indirect heat, cook the chicken breasts approximately 3 minutes on each side, giving a quarter turn on each side to create grill markings. Top the chicken breasts with the salsa.

Turkey Piccata

When you're running a little short on time, try this quick dish.

SERVES 4

1 pound boneless turkey breast, cut into ¼-inch diagonal
slices, or 1 pound turkey cutlets

Salt and freshly ground pepper

¼ cup all-purpose flour

1 large lemon

2 tablespoons olive oil

¼ cup dry white wine (optional)

½ cup low-fat, low-salt chicken stock

1 tablespoon drained capers

2 teaspoons unsalted butter

1 tablespoon chopped fresh parsley

Season the turkey slices on both sides with salt and pepper and dredge in flour, shaking off the excess. With a sharp paring knife, peel the lemon, removing all the white membrane. Cut segments from the peeled lemon, working over a bowl to catch any juice. Film a nonstick pan with the olive oil and cook the turkey slices 3 minutes on each side, until they are golden brown. Transfer the turkey to a plate to keep warm. Pour the white wine, if desired, into the pan and reduce by half, stirring constantly. Add the chicken stock, lemon segments and juice, and capers, bring to a boil, and cook 1 minute. Whisk in the butter and the parsley, check for seasoning, and spoon the sauce over the turkey slices.

Turkey Scallopini

Here's another way to use turkey cutlets.

SERVES 4

1 pound boneless turkey breast, cut into ¼-inch diagonal
    slices, or 1 pound turkey cutlets

Salt and freshly ground pepper

¼ cup all-purpose flour

2 tablespoons olive oil

1 cup sliced white mushrooms

1 teaspoon minced garlic

½ cup Marsala (optional)

½ cup well-drained diced canned tomatoes

½ cup low-fat, low-salt chicken stock

2 teaspoons unsalted butter

1 tablespoon chopped fresh parsley

Season the turkey slices on both sides with salt and pepper and dredge in flour, shaking off excess. Film a nonstick pan with the olive oil and cook the turkey slices 3 minutes on each side, until they are golden brown. Transfer the turkey to a plate to keep warm. In the same pan, sauté the mushrooms and garlic until they are softened, about 5 minutes. Add the Marsala, if desired, and bring to a boil, stirring constantly. Add the tomatoes and the chicken stock, bring to a boil, and cook 2 to 3 minutes, until the sauce reduces and thickens slightly. Whisk in the butter and the parsley, check for seasonings, and spoon the sauce over the turkey slices.

Paella

This is a great dish to serve when you want to impress company. Paella is traditionally served from the pan in which it is cooked, but you can also present it in a decorative serving dish.

Arborio is an Italian rice. If you can't find it in the rice section of your supermarket, try the international shelves or a gourmet market.

Cooked green beans or asparagus is also a nice addition to the paella.

SERVES 4

2 cups low-fat, low-sodium chicken broth

¼ teaspoon saffron threads or a pinch of powdered saffron

2 teaspoons olive oil

1 medium onion, chopped

2 teaspoons minced garlic

1 cup arborio rice

1 cup diced low-salt tomatoes with juice

Salt and freshly ground pepper

½ pound skinless, boneless chicken breast, cut into 1-inch strips

½ pound medium shrimp, peeled, deveined, and the tails left on

½ pound mussels, scrubbed and debearded

1 cup frozen baby artichoke hearts

1 cup frozen baby peas

1 roasted red bell pepper, jarred or homemade, peeled, seeded, and cut into thin strips

Combine the chicken broth and the saffron in a small saucepan and heat to simmer; set aside and keep warm. Film a large nonstick skillet with 1 teaspoon olive oil and heat to medium. Add the onion and garlic and cook for about 5 minutes, stirring, until softened. Add the arborio rice and stir to coat with the olive oil. You might need to add another teaspoon of olive oil. Add the tomatoes and stir well. Add the reserved saffron chicken broth, salt, and pepper, and cover, reduce heat to low, and cook for 20 minutes. After 20 minutes, stir in the chicken breast strips, the shrimp, and the mussels, cover, and cook 10 minutes more. Arrange the artichoke hearts, peas, and red pepper over the top, cover, and cook for a final 5 minutes. Correct seasoning. The Spanish allow the paella to "rest" for a few minutes to marry the flavors before serving.

Side Dishes

IF STEAMED VEGETABLES HAVE ALWAYS BEEN your idea of the only healthy side dish, I think you'll be pleasantly surprised to find that there are many other options. While, for instance, you might not have considered potato and coleslaw dishes appropriate choices—and the way they're usually prepared, they're not—the variations on those themes here can be eaten without guilt. Like the other side dishes coming up, they're as nutritious as they are delicious.

Healthy Coleslaw

This crunchy side salad will enhance any sandwich. I like it with my Portabella Mushroom Burger (page 156).

SERVES 4

½ cup light sour cream
½ cup light mayonnaise
2 tablespoons Dijon mustard
2 teaspoons honey
2 teaspoons red wine vinegar
½ head green cabbage, very thinly sliced
1 medium carrot, peeled and grated
1 red onion, halved and very thinly sliced
2 tablespoons currants
1 apple, cored, halved, and thinly sliced
Salt and freshly ground pepper

Combine the sour cream, mayonnaise, mustard, honey, and vinegar in a bowl. Add the shredded cabbage, carrot, onion, currants, and apple. Season with salt and pepper. Cover and set aside for 1 hour in the refrigerator, then taste. You may want to add more vinegar or salt.

Roasted Red Beets

You may want to double up on this recipe and keep them on hand. They are a very tasty addition to any salad and keep quite well in the refrigerator.

SERVES 4 TO 6

6 medium beets
2 tablespoons olive oil
2 tablespoons red wine vinegar
Salt and freshly ground pepper
A few sprigs of fresh thyme
1 small onion, sliced

Preheat the oven to 350°F. Scrub the beets with a vegetable brush and pat dry with a paper towel. Make an aluminum foil "packet" and place the beets inside. Drizzle with the olive oil and vinegar. Season with salt and pepper. Place a few sprigs of fresh thyme and a few slices of onion over the beets. Close and seal the packet by crimping the edges tightly. Place the packet on a baking sheet and put in the oven for 1 to 1½ hours. The cooking time will depend on the size of the beets. The beets are done when they can be pierced easily with a skewer. Cool the beets in their packet and, when cool, peel and slice them into thin wedges. Store the beets in a covered container in the refrigerator.

Zucchini with Cilantro and Yogurt

This cool vegetable dish is a fine accompaniment to spicy food.

SERVES 4

1 pound small to medium zucchini

1 inch fresh ginger root, peeled and grated

⅔ cup nonfat or low-fat plain yogurt

2 tablespoons coarsely chopped cilantro

Salt and freshly ground pepper

Wash the zucchini and slice into ½-inch rounds. Place the zucchini in a steamer basket over boiling water. Sprinkle the ginger over the zucchini, cover, and steam for 3 to 5 minutes. In a small saucepan, warm the yogurt with the cilantro, salt, and pepper. When the zucchini are tender-crisp, mix with the warmed yogurt, correct the seasoning, and serve.

Braised Swiss Chard with Raisins and Pine Nuts

These greens have an Italian flair. I like to get my Swiss chard from the farmers' market. This dish is also excellent made with spinach; use two bunches or ready-to-cook triple-washed packages from the supermarket.

SERVES 4

One large bunch Swiss chard
1 tablespoon olive oil
1 medium red onion, halved and thinly sliced
2 tablespoons golden or regular raisins or currants
2 tablespoons pine nuts
Salt and freshly ground pepper
¼ cup water
Red wine or balsamic vinegar (optional)

Wash the Swiss chard well. Remove the leaves from the stems and tear the leaves into medium-size pieces. Set aside. Place a large nonstick pan over medium-high heat and film the bottom with olive oil. Stir in the red onion and cook for about 5 minutes, until softened. Add the raisins and pine nuts and stir to toast the nuts. Now add the Swiss chard, give it a couple of stirs, add the water, and cover the pan to wilt the chard. This should take about 3 minutes. Season with salt and pepper. Divide among 4 plates. Add a splash of red wine or balsamic vinegar, if desired.

Summer Succotash

This super side dish takes advantage of summer's bounty. Try it at your next barbecue.

SERVES 4 TO 6

1 tablespoon olive oil

1 red onion, diced

1 clove garlic, minced

1 cup fresh yellow or white corn kernels

1 cup steamed green beans, cut on the diagonal into 1-inch pieces

1 medium zucchini, diced

2 medium red pepper, seeded and diced

½ cup fresh or frozen baby peas or snap peas (optional)

½ cup low-fat, low-salt chicken stock

Salt and freshly ground pepper

Place a nonstick pan over medium-high heat and film with the olive oil. Add the onion and garlic and cook until softened, stirring occasionally, for 3 to 5 minutes. Do not brown. Add the corn, green beans, zucchini, pepper, and peas (if using) to the pan, and stir well. Add the chicken stock. Cover the pan and cook about 5 minutes, until the vegetables are cooked through. Season with salt and pepper.

Mashed Potatoes

I like to use Yukon Gold potatoes for this recipe. These potatoes have a very buttery, rich flavor, so you don't need butter or a lot of salt. If you can't find Yukon Golds at your supermarket, use russet potatoes instead.

SERVES 4

4 large Yukon Gold potatoes, peeled and cut into large
    chunks
Salt
1 to 1½ cups hot 1 percent milk
2 tablespoons light sour cream
1 teaspoon chopped garlic
Freshly ground pepper

Place the potatoes in a pot and cover with cold water. Salt the water and bring to a boil. Cook the potatoes until done, about 15 to 20 minutes. Drain the potatoes in a colander, then place in the bowl of an electric mixer fitted with a wire whip attachment. Beat at medium speed to break up the potatoes, then add the hot milk, sour cream and chopped garlic. Scrape down the side with a rubber spatula to break up any lumps and whip for 1 minute on high speed. Season with salt and pepper to taste and serve hot.

Small Rustic Roasted Red Potatoes

This is one of my favorite ways to eat potatoes. Not only is this dish delicious, the roasting herbs make your kitchen smell wonderful.

SERVES 4

16 to 20 small red potatoes, all of uniform size

2 tablespoons olive oil

Kosher salt and fresh ground pepper

A few fresh thyme or rosemary branches

Preheat oven to 350°F. Spread the potatoes in a single layer on a non-stick baking sheet. Drizzle the potatoes with olive oil and sprinkle with kosher salt and pepper. Use your hands to roll the potatoes around on the baking sheet to ensure that they are all coated with olive oil. Lay the herb branches over the potatoes and roast for 20 to 30 minutes, depending on the size of the potatoes. Discard herb branches after cooking.

Oven-Baked Steak "Fries"

Healthful eating does not mean life without "fries." I think you'll be surprised at how terrific these low-fat non-fried fries are.

SERVES 4

Nonfat cooking spray

2 tablespoons olive oil

1 teaspoon chopped garlic

1 tablespoon water

Juice of one lemon

½ teaspoon paprika

Dash of cayenne pepper

1 tablespoon chopped fresh rosemary

Salt and freshly ground pepper

2 large russet potatoes, cut the potato in half lengthwise. Then cut into wedges that are ½ inch wide at the widest end.

Preheat the oven to 400°F. Spray a nonstick baking sheet with cooking spray. In a medium mixing bowl, combine the olive oil, garlic, water, lemon juice, paprika, cayenne pepper, rosemary, salt, and pepper. Toss a few of the potato wedges at a time in the mixing bowl, coating each wedge evenly. Arrange in one layer on the baking sheet and bake for 25 to 30 minutes until browned, turning the pan once or twice to ensure even browning.

Maple Glazed and Roasted Yams

Don't wait for Thanksgiving to try these. And be sure you use real maple syrup!

SERVES 4

2 tablespoons maple syrup
2 tablespoons olive oil or canola oil
4 medium-size yams
Kosher salt and freshly ground pepper

Preheat oven to 350°F. In a small bowl, combine the maple syrup and oil. Scrub the yams with a vegetable brush and pat dry with a paper towel. Slice the yams in half lengthwise and rub the cut surface with the maple syrup/oil mix. Place the yams on a foil- or parchment-lined baking sheet and sprinkle with salt and pepper. Tent the yams loosely with another sheet of aluminum foil and bake for 25 minutes. Remove foil, baste again with the maple syrup/oil mixture, and cook uncovered for another 20 to 25 minutes. If you have any leftover glaze, baste every 10 minutes. When done, remove from oven and cool until you are able to slip off the skins.

Wild Mushroom Grits

Grits aren't just for breakfast anymore!

SERVES 4

3 tablespoons olive oil

2 cups mixed sliced mushrooms (button, shiitake, portabella, morels, chanterelles—whatever is available)

1 large shallot, diced

3 cups nonfat milk

3 cups low-fat, low-salt chicken stock or water

1 cup medium-ground white grits

4 tablespoons Parmesan cheese

Salt and freshly ground pepper

1 tablespoon chopped parsley or chives, for garnish

Place a medium nonstick skillet over medium-high heat. Add the olive oil, then the sliced mushrooms and shallot. Cook, stirring often, until the shallots are softened and mushrooms are cooked through, about 5 minutes. Set aside the mushrooms and keep warm. In a medium saucepan, bring the milk and chicken stock to a boil. Whisk in the grits, a handful at a time. Reduce the heat to medium and stir constantly until the grits are thick and creamy, about 15 minutes. Remove from heat and stir in the Parmesan cheese and season to taste with salt and pepper. Pour the grits into a serving dish. Top with the reserved mushrooms and their juices. Sprinkle with chopped parsley or chives.

Quinoa Pilaf

Quinoa, an ancient American grain, is a nutritional powerhouse with more protein than any other grain, high in unsaturated fats and low in carbohydrates. It can be found in most health food stores and many well-stocked supermarkets.

SERVES 4

1 tablespoon olive oil

1 carrot, peeled and diced

1 stalk celery, diced

1 small onion, diced

1 teaspoon chopped garlic

1 cup quinoa, well rinsed

1 bay leaf

Salt and freshly ground pepper

2 cups low-fat chicken stock or water

½ cup defrosted baby peas

Place a saucepan over medium-high heat. Add the olive oil and then the carrot, celery, onion, and garlic. Cook 5 to 7 minutes, stirring often, until the vegetables are softened but not browned. Add the rinsed quinoa, bay leaf, and salt and pepper, and stir to combine. Add the chicken stock or water and bring to a boil. Reduce to a simmer, cover the pot, and cook for 15 to 20 minutes, or until the liquid is absorbed. Fluff the grains with a fork and stir in the defrosted baby peas. Correct the seasonings and serve.

Black Beans

Try these with brown rice, warm corn tortillas, salsa, and lime wedges for a delicious vegetarian dinner, or use them to accompany Grilled Skinless Chicken Breasts with Mango-Tomato Salsa (page 181).

SERVES 6 TO 8

1 pound black beans, well washed and soaked overnight

1 tablespoon olive oil

1 onion, chopped

1 tablespoon chopped garlic

2 stalks celery, diced

1 serrano chile, chopped (more if you like spicy food)

1 bay leaf

1 tablespoon toasted ground cumin

1 can dark beer (or cheap beer)

1 quart or more low-fat, low-salt chicken broth

Salt and freshly ground pepper

Drain the soaked beans and set aside. Place a large soup pot over medium-high heat. Add 1 tablespoon of olive oil and sauté the onion, garlic, celery, and chile until softened but not browned, about 5 minutes. Add the beans, bay leaf, and cumin. Add the beer, if desired, and chicken broth. Bring to a boil, reduce to a simmer, and cook until beans are soft, adding more liquid if necessary. This will take about an hour. Add salt and pepper to taste and ladle into shallow bowls.

Desserts

THE WORD "DESSERT" CONJURES UP VISIONS of high-calorie splurges that offer intense flavor but little in the way of nutrition. In fact, dessert doesn't have to be a throwaway dish. Many desserts can provide the sweetness and indulgence you crave along with something else, be it vitamins and minerals from fruit or even some protein from nuts or egg whites. These treats are great rewards for working hard to change your eating behavior, and they don't take you off the program. Instead, they fit right into your healthy way of life.

Cool Strawberries

This treat makes it worth the wait for local strawberries to come into season.

SERVES 4

1 large basket ripe organic strawberries
Sugar to taste
A few drops fresh lemon juice
1 pint of the best strawberry sorbet you can find
Mint spring for garnish
Orange liqueur, such as Triple Sec (optional)

Rinse and drain the strawberries. Thinly slice the berries into a bowl and lightly sprinkle them with sugar and lemon juice. Set aside for ½ hour so that the juices form a natural syrup. Divide the strawberries among four elegant dessert glasses, top with a small scoop of strawberry sorbet, and garnish with a mint sprig. Sprinkle each serving with a few drops of orange liqueur, if desired.

Chilled Fruit Soup with Frozen Vanilla Yogurt

A great, refreshing summer time dessert! You must use the ripest, most flavorful fruit you can find for this treat.

SERVES 4

1 large ripe cantaloupe

¼ cup fresh-squeezed orange juice

Juice of one large lemon

3 or 4 large ripe nectarines

3 tablespoons orange liqueur (optional)

Sugar to taste

Frozen vanilla yogurt

Cut the melon in half, discard the seeds and remove the skin with a sharp knife. Cut the melon into rough chunks. Place in a blender jar with the orange and lemon juice. Slice the nectarines and add to the blender. Puree all of the fruit at medium speed until it is a smooth liquid. Pour into a bowl and add the orange liqueur, if desired, and sweeten to taste. Chill for at least 3 to 4 hours. Ladle into four festive clear glass bowls and top with a scoop of frozen vanilla yogurt. Garnish with a sprig of mint.

Warm Apple Crisp

There's no better fall or winter dessert than a warm apple crisp. This would be delicious with a drizzle of plain nonfat yogurt sweetened with a little honey and a drop of pure vanilla extract, or a scoop of frozen vanilla yogurt.

SERVES 4

Nonfat cooking spray

2 cups peeled, cored and thinly sliced apples, such as
  Granny Smiths

2 tablespoons sugar, or to taste

¼ cup apple juice

1 tablespoon fresh lemon juice

2 teaspoons cornstarch

1 teaspoon ground cinnamon

Pinch of nutmeg

OAT TOPPING

½ cup walnuts or almonds, finely chopped

½ cup old-fashioned rolled oats

½ cup brown sugar

2 tablespoons all-purpose flour

2 tablespoons softened unsalted butter

Preheat the oven to 350°F. Coat an 8-inch-square shallow baking dish with cooking spray.

In a large bowl, toss together the apples, sugar, apple juice, lemon juice, cornstarch, cinnamon, and nutmeg until well combined. Set aside.

MAKE THE OATMEAL TOPPING:

In the bowl of an electric mixer fitted with a paddle, gently combine the walnuts or almonds, oats, brown sugar, flour, and butter at low speed.

Place the apple mixture in the dish. Sprinkle the topping evenly over the apples and bake for 25 to 30 minutes, until the apples are cooked through, the juices are bubbling, and the topping is browned. Serve hot, warm, or at room temperature.

Poached Pears

This versatile recipe is worthy of being served at your most elegant dinner parties.

SERVES 4

4 medium-size pears, peeled, halved and cored
1 cup apple juice
1 cinnamon stick
¼ cup honey
¼ cup sugar
1 teaspoon pure vanilla extract
1 bay leaf
1 cup white wine (optional)
1 lemon, cut in half

Place the pears in a nonreactive saucepan. Add the apple juice, cinnamon stick, honey, sugar, vanilla, bay leaf, and white wine, if desired, to the pan. Squeeze the juice from the lemon into the pan and add the halves to the pan. Bring the pears to a simmer. Cover with a round of waxed paper or parchment and simmer until the pears are soft but still retain their shape, about 20 to 25 minutes. Remove the cinnamon stick and bay leaf and allow the pears to cool in their cooking liquid.

Poached Pears with Topping

A perfect topping for a perfect dessert!

SERVES 4

Nonfat cooking spray
1 recipe Poached Pears (page 206)
1 recipe Oat Topping from Warm Apple Crisp (page 204)
Nonfat vanilla yogurt

Preheat the broiler. Spray a shallow baking dish with cooking spray. Place the warm pear halves in the dish, cut side up, and top each half with one tablespoon of the Oat Topping. Broil until the topping is browned, about 3 minutes. Place 2 pear halves on each plate and drizzle yogurt over all.

Warm Poached Pear and Dried Fruit Compote

So rich in flavor and so good for you! Serve this with biscotti or amaretti (Italian almond cookies) on the side.

SERVES 4

1 recipe Poached Pears (page 206)
8 dried apricot halves
4 dried pitted prunes
1 cup golden raisins

Prepare the pears as instructed in the recipe. Remove the pears from the poaching liquid and add the dried apricots, prunes, and raisins. Simmer a few minutes, until the dried fruits are plumped. Divide the pears among four bowls and spoon the poached dried fruit and some of the syrup over each serving.

Goat Cheese with Honey and Nuts

Instead of cookies or cake, try this elegant cheese course to end your meal.

SERVES 4

1 4-ounce log of fresh goat cheese, cut into 4 rounds,
   at room temperature

2 tablespoons good honey

4 tablespoons toasted walnuts or almonds

4 slices toasted French baguette

4 sprigs of fresh thyme, for garnish

Cut the goat cheese into rounds and place each one in the middle of a small serving plate. Drizzle the cheese with honey and surround each round with the walnuts or almonds. Serve with a slice of toasted baquette and garnish with a sprig of fresh thyme.

Afogato

Afogato is traditionally made with a scoop of vanilla ice cream served in a coffee cup with a dose of espresso poured over it. This more healthful version uses vanilla or caramel yogurt. If you're cutting back on caffeine, try it with decaffeinated espresso.

MAKES 1 SERVING

1 scoop frozen vanilla or caramel yogurt
1 cup regular or decaffeinated espresso
Toasted walnuts or almonds, for garnish

Place a scoop of frozen yogurt in a coffee cup (or dish) and pour a serving of espresso on top. Sprinkle with the toasted nuts and serve immediately.

Panna Cotta

Panna Cotta is a simple eggless custard flavored with lemon zest. It goes well with fresh fruit or, in the winter, with dried fruit compote. You could also try it with Raspberry Sauce (page 216).

SERVES 4

Nonfat cooking spray
½ package unflavored gelatin
1 cup low-fat milk
1 cup evaporated skim milk
½ cup sugar
Zest of ½ lemon
1-inch piece vanilla bean, split, or 1 teaspoon pure vanilla
   extract

Spray four 6-ounce custard cups with cooking spray and place in the refrigerator to chill. Soften the gelatin by placing 1½ tablespoons cold water in a small bowl. Sprinkle the gelatin over the water and set aside. Place the milks, sugar, lemon zest, and vanilla bean in a small saucepan and heat to a simmer.

Remove the pan from the heat and scrape the split vanilla bean with a paring knife to remove the seeds. Return the seeds to the milk mixture and discard the pod. Cool the milk, stirring occasionally. When the milk is about the temperature of hot tap water, add ½ cup milk to the softened gelatin, stirring until the gelatin is completely dissolved. Add the remaining 1½ cups milk and stir well. Divide among the four chilled custard cups and refrigerate overnight.

Unmold the Panna Cotta by running a knife around the edges and invert onto serving plates (tap to loosen).

Pavlova

This crisp meringue base topped with fresh fruit, frozen yogurt, and a fruit sauce is a famous Australian dessert; it is named after the Russian ballerina Anna Pavlova.

During the fall and winter, when berries aren't in season, Pavlova can be made with tropical fruits, such as pineapple, kiwifruit, passion fruit, or mango.

Don't try to make this on a hot, humid day; the meringues won't get as crisp as they should.

MAKES FOUR 4-INCH MERINGUE SHELLS
OR ONE 9-INCH ROUND

4 egg whites
1 teaspoon pure vanilla extract
Pinch of cream of tartar
1 cup granulated sugar
Vanilla frozen yogurt
1 pint mixed berries (strawberries, raspberries, blueberries, blackberries—whatever is available)
Sifted confectioners' sugar, for garnish
Raspberry Sauce (page 216)

Preheat the oven to 250°F. Place the egg whites in the bowl of an electric mixer. Beat until foamy; add the vanilla extract and cream of tartar. Continue to beat at high speed while gradually adding the sugar. Beat until stiff peaks form, but do not overbeat or the egg whites will be grainy. Fill a pastry bag fitted with a plain tip with the beaten egg whites and pipe onto a parchment-lined baking sheet, forming individual meringues of 4-inch circles or one large 9-inch circle. This can also be done with a spoon by dropping dollops of meringue onto the parchment-lined baking sheet and smoothing them into shape with the back of the spoon. Cook for 1 hour or longer, depending on the size, until the meringues are stiff but not browned. Turn the oven off, open the door, and let the meringues cool gradually. If you're not going to use the meringues immediately, store them in an airtight container.

If serving individual meringues, set each shell on a plate. Place a small scoop of frozen yogurt in the center of each shell and divide the berries equally over the tops. Sprinkle with confectioners' sugar and top with Raspberry Sauce.

If serving one large meringue, place the shell on a serving plate. Place 4 small scoops of vanilla frozen yogurt in the center of the shell, cover the shell with the berries, and lightly sprinkle with confectioners' sugar. Cut the meringue shell into four wedges, making sure each portion has a scoop of yogurt and a portion of berries. Pass the Raspberry Sauce!

Chocolate Almond Angel Food Cake

This luscious cake is as light as a feather and full of chocolate flavor—and contains almost no fat. Make sure that your bowl and beaters are absolutely clean and grease-free and there's not a speck of yolk in your egg whites; fold the whites gently into the flour mixture to make sure you get maximum volume.

Serve the cake with Raspberry Sauce (page 216), fresh fruit of your choice, or a small scoop of caramel-flavored frozen yogurt.

MAKES ONE 10-INCH CAKE

¾ cup cake flour

¼ cup unsweetened cocoa powder (not Dutch process)

Pinch of salt

1 cup sugar

12 egg whites, at room temperature

1 teaspoon cream of tartar

1 teaspoon pure vanilla extract

⅓ cup blanched toasted almonds, finely chopped

Raspberry Sauce (optional)

Sliced fresh fruit or berries (optional)

Caramel frozen yogurt (optional)

Position the oven rack in the lower third of the oven. Preheat the oven to 350°F. Sift together the flour, cocoa powder, salt, and ¼ cup of the sugar and set aside. In a clean, dry bowl of an electric mixer, beat the egg whites until foamy. Add the cream of tartar, and vanilla extract and continue to beat at high speed, gradually adding the remaining ¾ cup sugar. Beat just until stiff peaks form; do not over-beat, or the whites will become grainy. Sift ¼ of the flour mixture over the beaten egg whites and gently fold it into the whites with a rubber spatula. Alternately fold in the almonds and the remaining flour mixture in small batches, until everything is just incorporated. Pour the batter into an *ungreased* 10-inch tube pan, run a spatula through the mixture to remove any air pockets, and smooth the top. Bake for 45 to 50 minutes, until a toothpick inserted in the middle of the cake comes out clean. Remove the cake from the oven and invert the pan over an upended funnel or bottle. Allow the cake to cool completely, about 1 hour. Run a knife around the edges of the pan and the tube to loosen the cake and turn it onto a serving platter.

Raspberry Sauce

This makes a great topping for frozen yogurt or fresh berries, and really dresses up the Chocolate Almond Angel Food Cake (page 214) and Pavlova (page 212). It's just as good made with frozen unsweetened raspberries as it is with fresh, which means it's a year-round treat. The sauce will keep, tightly covered, for five days in the refrigerator.

MAKES ABOUT 2 CUPS

3 cups fresh raspberries or 1 package thawed, unsweetened
   frozen raspberries
⅓ cup sugar
1 tablespoon lemon juice
1 tablespoon orange liqueur or port wine (optional)

In a blender, puree the raspberries, sugar, lemon juice, and liqueur, if desired. Strain the sauce through a fine-mesh sieve to remove any seeds. Store in the refrigerator until needed.

Spicy Toasted Walnuts

The egg white makes these nuts crisp beautifully, and the cayenne pepper gives them a nice flavor zip. You could also try other seasonings, such as cinnamon or curry powder. Try them sprinkled over a salad, over nonfat yogurt, or as a snack. Store the nuts in an airtight jar.

MAKES ABOUT 2 CUPS

2 cups raw walnut halves
1 egg white, lightly beaten
Salt
1 tablespoon sugar
½ teaspoon cayenne pepper, or to taste
Nonfat cooking spray (optional)

Preheat the oven to 350°F. Put the walnuts in a bowl, add the egg white, and toss very well to coat the nuts evenly. Sprinkle with the salt, sugar, and cayenne pepper and toss some more. Spread the walnuts on a nonstick baking sheet or one sprayed with nonfat cooking spray. Toast the walnuts in for 8 to 10 minutes, turning the pan several times to ensure even roasting. Remove the sheet from the oven and let the nuts cool completely before using or storing.

Index

aerobic exercise, 7–8, 9, 13–14, 18–21
Afogato, 210
aging process, 24
alcohol, 17, 72–73, 97–98
amino acids, 72
antioxidants, 56, 63, 64, 73, 74, 80, 83, 84
appetizers, 99
apples
  Bran Muffins with Fruit, 110
  Crispy Romaine Salad with Apples, Celery, Toasted Walnuts, and Light Blue Cheese Dressing, 137
  Warm Apple Crisp, 204–5
  Wild Rice Salad, 142–43
apricots, Warm Poached Pear and Dried Fruit Compote, 208
artichokes
  Artichoke and Tuna Panini, 159
  Lemon Parsley Chicken Breast with Baby Artichokes and Potatoes, 180
  Paella, 184–85
asparagus
  Asparagus Vinaigrette, 138
  Tuna with Grape Tomatoes and Greens, 144
  Vegetable Frittata, 164
aspirin, 73
Atkins diet, 2–3
attitude check, 14–15, 57
avocado, Spicy Mexican Shrimp Cocktail, 149–50

Baby Greens with Warm Goat Cheese and Walnut Vinaigrette, 135–36
Baked Lemon Herb Halibut, 176
bananas
  Bran Muffins with Fruit, 110
  Fresh Fruit Medley, 107
  Peaches and "Cream" Fresh Fruit Smoothie, 106
basil, recipes for, 139, 140, 170–71
B complex, 74–75, 81
beans, green
  Green Bean Salad with Toasted Walnuts, 141
  Provençal Vegetable Soup (Soupe au Pistou), 128–29
  Salade Niçoise, 145–46
  Summer Succotash, 192

beans, legumes, 72
    Black Beans, 199
    Curried Lentil Soup with Yogurt, 130
    Hummus with Toasted Pita Triangles, 151–52
    Pan-Seared Fillet of Tilapia with Mango Tomato Salsa and Lentil Pancake, 172–73
    Provençal Vegetable Soup (Soupe au Pistou), 128–29
    Red Bean Soup, 131
    Tuna with Grape Tomatoes and Greens, 144
beets
    Roasted Red Beets, 189
    Salade Niçoise, 145–46
berries, 84
    Blueberry Buttermilk Pancakes, 111–12
    Cool Strawberries, 202
    Granola Yogurt Parfait, 109
    Pavlova, 212–13
    Raspberry Sauce, 216
beta-carotene, 56, 64, 75, 83
bingeing, 43–44, 100, 101–2
Black Beans, 199
blood sugar (glucose), 30–31, 37, 51, 61, 66–68
blueberries. See berries
bok choy, Tofu and Broccoli Stir Fry, 162–63
boredom, 22, 45, 48, 49, 56, 90
Braised Swiss Chard with Raisins and Pine Nuts, 191
Bran Muffins with Fruit, 110
bread
    avoiding, 98
    sandwich recipes, 154–59
    whole-grain, 77, 82, 93, 110, 178
    See also grains, whole
Bread Crumbs, Quick Herbed, 178

breakfast, 29–40
    composition of, 35–38, 39
    energy levels and, 30–31
    exercise and, 35–37, 39–40
    hunger and, 31, 32–33
    ideas for, 38–39
    importance of, 33–35, 59
    metabolism and, 30, 32
    quality of, 37–38
    recipes for, 105–18
    sample meals, 54
    size of, 31, 37
    timing of, 34–37, 39–40
broccoli, 83
    Broccoli and Swiss Chard Cannelloni, 166–67
    Tofu and Broccoli Stir Fry, 162–63
bulgur wheat, 93
butternut squash, Gingered Butternut Squash Soup, 124

cabbage, Healthy Coleslaw, 188
caffeine, 17, 38, 60
Cake, Chocolate Almond Angel Food, 214–15
calcium, 56, 75, 83
calories
    in alcohol, 73
    breakfast and, 31, 37
    in carbohydrates, 61, 73
    daily consumption of, 58–59
    distribution of, 37, 50–54, 59
    energy levels and, 50, 51, 52
    in fats, 61, 69, 73
    in snacks during day, 49–50, 53
Cambridge diet, 4
cancer, 4, 6, 42, 63, 72, 73, 80
canola oil, 70, 76, 84
carbohydrates, 60–66
    at breakfast, 35–37, 39
    calories per gram, 61, 73
    defined, 60–61

carbohydrates (*cont.*)
  as fuel, 71
  glycogen, 3, 20, 35, 61, 71–72
  starchy foods, 61, 64
  sugars, 61, 65–66, 67, 76–78
  very-low-carbohydrate, high-
    protein approach, 2–4, 5, 6
  whole grains, 37–38, 62, 64–65
carbonated water, 17
celery, Crispy Romaine Salad with
    Apples, Celery, Toasted Walnuts,
    and Light Blue Cheese Dressing,
    137
cereals, 37–38, 77, 92
  Granola Yogurt Parfait, 109
  Homemade Granola, 108
  See also grains, whole; *names of
    specific grains*
chamomile tea, 38, 44–45, 48
cheese
  Baby Greens with Warm Goat
    Cheese and Walnut Vinaigrette,
    135–36
  Broccoli and Swiss Chard
    Cannelloni, 166–67
  Crispy Romaine Salad with
    Apples, Celery, Toasted Walnuts,
    and Light Blue Cheese Dressing,
    137
  Fresh Summer Tomato Salad with
    Fresh Mozzarella and Basil, 139
  Goat Cheese with Honey and
    Nuts, 209
  Portabella Mushroom Burgers,
    156–57
  See also dairy products
chickpeas. *See* beans, legumes
Chilled Fruit Soup with Frozen
    Vanilla Yogurt, 203
Chocolate Almond Angel Food Cake,
    214–15
cholesterol, 64, 69, 80, 82–83

cilantro, Zucchini with Cilantro and
    Yogurt, 190
coffee, 17, 38, 60
Compote, Warm Poached Pear and
    Dried Fruit, 208
Cool Strawberries, 202
corn
  Corn Chowder, 126–27
  Summer Succotash, 192
corn syrup, 65, 76, 78
couscous, 93
  Tomatoes Stuffed with Couscous,
    Cucumber, and Mint, 153
Crispy Romaine Salad with Apples,
    Celery, Toasted Walnuts, and
    Light Blue Cheese Dressing, 137
cucumber
  Spicy Mexican Shrimp Cocktail,
    149–50
  Tomatoes Stuffed with Couscous,
    Cucumber, and Mint, 153
Curried Lentil Soup with Yogurt,
    130

dairy products, 63, 78
  Afogato, 210
  Blueberry Buttermilk Pancakes,
    111–12
  Chilled Fruit Soup with Frozen
    Vanilla Yogurt, 203
  Corn Chowder, 126–27
  Curried Lentil Soup with Yogurt,
    130
  Fresh Fruit Medley, 107
  Gingered Butternut Squash Soup,
    124
  Granola Yogurt Parfait, 109
  Leek and Potato Soup, 125
  Mashed Potatoes, 193
  Mushroom Soup, 122–23
  Panna Cotta, 211
  Pavlova, 212–13

Peaches and "Cream" Fresh Fruit
Smoothie, 106
Roasted Tomato Soup, 120
Wild Mushroom Grits, 197
Zucchini with Cilantro and
Yogurt, 190
See also cheese
dehydration, 16–17, 53–55
depression, 23
deprivation, 56, 102
desserts
dining out, 100
recipes for, 201–15
diabetes, 23
diet drugs, 5–6
diets, fad, 1–6
dining out, 95–100
dinner
sample meals, 54–55
size of, 51–53
drugs, diet, 5–6

edamame, 81
Eggplant and Zucchini Poor Boy
Sandwich, 154
eggs/egg whites, 72, 82–83
Asparagus Vinaigrette, 138
Breakfast Fried Rice (With or
Without Rice), 118
Chocolate Almond Angel Food
Cake, 214–15
Pavlova, 212–13
Poached Eggs with Veggie Hash,
116–17
Potato Omelet, 115
Salade Niçoise, 145–46
Scrambled Egg Whites with
Spinach and Orange, 114
Vegetable Frittata, 164
See also protein
emotional eating, 7, 9, 22–24
bingeing, 43–44, 100, 101–2

journals and, 23–24, 47, 49
nature of, 21–22
overcoming, 22–24, 59, 101–2
snacks and, 44–46, 53
energy levels, 30–31, 37, 41–42,
50–54
enzymes, 19
espresso, Afogato, 210
excuses, 14
exercise
aerobic, 7–8, 9, 13–14, 18–21
alcohol and, 73
as alternative to eating, 24
attitudes toward, 57
carbohydrates and, 71
discomfort of, 46
hydration during, 17
importance of, 7, 13–14, 15,
59
machines, 6, 19
metabolism and, 7–8, 9, 13–14
strength training, 7–8, 9, 13–14,
24–26, 72
timing of, 35–37, 39–40

fad diets, 1–6
farmers' markets, 85–87
fat
aerobic exercise and, 19–21
calories per gram, 61, 69, 73
in diet, 2–3, 4–5, 46–48, 61, 64,
67–70, 76, 82
fat-free foods, 5, 68–69, 78
percentage of total daily calories,
69
storage of body, 50, 51, 52, 59, 66,
71
Fen-phen, 5
fiber, 61, 64, 68
filters, water, 18
fish. See seafood and fish
flaxseed, 70, 84

food choices, 56–75
food shopping, 84–90
free-range products, 94
Fresh Fruit Medley, 107
Fresh Summer Tomato Salad with
    Fresh Mozzarella and Basil,
    139
fried foods, 64, 70
fructose, 65, 76, 77
fruit
    berries, 84
    at breakfast, 37–38
    daily servings of, 63–64, 67
    dessert and, 100
    farmers' markets and,
        85–87
    glycemic index and, 68
    serving size, 62
    sweet tooth and, 66
    tips for buying, 90–92
    See also names of specific fruits
Fruity Green Salad, 134

garlic, *Pistou,* 129
Gingered Butternut Squash Soup,
    124
glucose (blood sugar), 30–31, 37, 51,
    61, 66–68
glycemic index, 66–68
glycerol, 69
glycogen, 3, 20, 35, 61, 71–72
Goat Cheese with Honey and Nuts,
    209
gout, 3
grains, whole, 37–38, 62, 64–65, 67,
    68, 72, 77, 82
    recipes for, 107–12, 118, 142–43,
        168–69, 174–75, 197, 198,
        204–5, 207
    tips for buying, 92–94
    See also bread; pasta, whole-wheat;
        names of specific grains

granola
    Granola Yogurt Parfait, 109
    Homemade, 108
green beans. *See* beans, green
Grilled Skinless Chicken Breasts with
    Mango-Tomato Salsa, 181
Grilled Tuna or Swordfish with
    Roasted Red Pepper Vinaigrette,
    179
"Grilled" Veggie Burgers, 155
grocery shopping, 84–90

habit
    of eating breakfast, 33–35, 59
    of late-night snacks, 44–46
health food stores, 87, 88–89
Healthy Coleslaw, 188
heart
    cardiovascular fitness and,
        18–21
    problems with, 3, 4, 5, 69, 70, 73,
        80
    target heart range, 20–21
herbal tea, 38, 44–45, 48
Hoisin Shrimp and Okra with Brown
    Rice, 174–75
Homemade Granola, 108
Hummus with Toasted Pita
    Triangles, 151–52
hunger, 22–23
    "artificial," 53–55
    at breakfast, 31, 32–33
    calories and, 58
    discomfort of, 46–48
    late-night snacks and, 31, 40,
        41–42
hydration, 9, 16–18, 59, 60
hydrogenated fats, 69, 82

insulin shock, large meals and, 37, 51,
    66–67, 68
Internet shopping, 89–90

journals, 23–24, 47, 49
juice, 76, 98

ketones, 3
kidney health, 3, 71
kiwifruit
    Fresh Fruit Medley, 107
    Peaches and "Cream" Fresh Fruit
        Smoothie, 106

labels, food, 78, 89, 94
late-night snacks, 21, 22, 31, 40–49,
    59
leafy greens, 83, 91–92. *See also*
    salads; *names of specific greens*
leeks
    Fish Chowder, 132
    Leek and Potato Soup, 125
legumes. *See* beans, legumes
lemons
    Baked Lemon Herb Halibut,
        176
    Citrus Vinaigrette, 142–43
    Lemon Parsley Chicken Breast
        with Baby Artichokes and
        Potatoes, 180
lentils
    Curried Lentil Soup with Yogurt,
        130
    Pan-Seared Fillet of Tilapia with
        Mango Tomato Salsa and Lentil
        Pancake, 172–73
liquid diets, 4
liver health, 3, 71
loneliness, 22
lunch, 54

mangos
    Fresh Fruit Medley, 107
    Grilled Skinless Chicken Breasts
        with Mango-Tomato Salsa,
        181

Pan-Seared Fillet of Tilapia with
    Mango Tomato Salsa and Lentil
    Pancake, 172–73
Maple Glazed and Roasted Yams, 196
Marinara Sauce, 167
Marinated Italian Seafood Salad,
    147–48
Mashed Potatoes, 193
meat
    processed, 78
    serving size, 62–63
    tips for buying, 94
    See also protein
melon, Chilled Fruit Soup with
    Frozen Vanilla Yogurt, 203
metabolism, 15–26
    aerobic exercise and, 7–8, 9
    alcohol and, 73
    calories and, 50
    hydration and, 16–18, 60
    sign of slow, 32
    sleep and, 15–16, 30, 41, 51
    snacks and, 53
    strength training and, 7–8, 9,
        13–14
    timing of meals and, 30, 32, 35–37,
        39–40, 50
micronutrients, 63
milk. *See* dairy products
minerals, 55, 74
mint, Tomatoes Stuffed with
    Couscous, Cucumber, and Mint,
    153
monounsaturated fats, 69–70, 76,
    79–80
multivitamins, 74
mushrooms, 81
    Breakfast Fried Rice (With or
        Without Rice), 118
    Mushroom Soup, 122–23
    Polenta with Swiss Chard and
        Portabella Mushrooms, 168–69

mushrooms (*cont.*)
  Portabella Mushroom Burgers,
    156–57
  Tofu and Broccoli Stir Fry, 162–63
  Turkey Scallopini, 183
  Vegetable Frittata, 164
  Wild Mushroom Grits, 197
Mustard-Crusted Baked Salmon,
    177–78

natural food supermarkets, 87–88
nectarines, Chilled Fruit Soup with
    Frozen Vanilla Yogurt, 203
nutrients, 59–75
  calorie levels and, 58–59
  carbohydrates, 60–66, 71–72
  defined, 59
  dining out, 96
  fat, 2–3, 4–5, 46–48, 61, 67–70, 76,
    79–80, 82
  fiber, 61, 64, 68
  fruits, 37–38, 62, 63–64, 67
  glycemic index, 66–68
  labels and, 78, 89, 94
  protein, 68, 70–72
  serving sizes, 62–63
  sugar, 61, 65–66, 76, 77, 78
  supplements, 55, 73–75
  vegetables, 62, 63–64, 67
  water, 59–60, 76–77
  whole grains, 37–38, 62, 64–65, 72,
    77, 92–94
nuts, 72, 81–82
  Afogato, 210
  Braised Swiss Chard with Raisins
    and Pine Nuts, 191
  Chocolate Almond Angel Food
    Cake, 214–15
  Crispy Romaine Salad with
    Apples, Celery, Toasted Walnuts,
    and Light Blue Cheese Dressing,
    137

Goat Cheese with Honey and
    Nuts, 209
  Granola Yogurt Parfait, 109
  Green Bean Salad with Toasted
    Walnuts, 141
  Homemade Granola, 108
  Poached Pears with Topping, 207
  Spicy Toasted Walnuts, 217
  Warm Apple Crisp, 204–5
  Wild Rice Salad, 142–43

oats, 64, 68, 77, 92
  Granola Yogurt Parfait, 109
  Homemade Granola, 108
  Poached Pears with Topping, 207
  Warm Apple Crisp, 204–5
obesity, 4, 76
okra, Hoisin Shrimp and Okra with
    Brown Rice, 174–75
olive oil, 69–70, 76, 79–80
omega-3 fatty acids, 70, 83–84
Optifast diet, 4
oranges
  Chilled Fruit Soup with Frozen
    Vanilla Yogurt, 203
  Scrambled Egg Whites with
    Spinach and Orange, 114
organic foods, 86–87, 94
osteoporosis, 75
Oven-Baked Steak "Fries," 195

Paella, 184–85
pancakes
  Blueberry Buttermilk Pancakes,
    111–12
  Lentil, 172–73
  Potato Pancakes, 113
Panna Cotta, 211
Pan-Seared Fillet of Tilapia with
    Mango Tomato Salsa and Lentil
    Pancake, 172–73
papaya, Fresh Fruit Medley, 107

pasta, whole-wheat, 93, 94
  Broccoli and Swiss Chard
    Cannelloni, 166–67
  Provençal Vegetable Soup *(Soupe
    au Pistou)*, 128–29
  Spinach Penne with Spicy Roasted
    Pepper Sauce, 165
  Steamed Manila Clams and
    Mussels in White Wine Broth
    with Chili Flakes and Spaghetti,
    170–71
  Tomatoes Stuffed with Couscous,
    Cucumber, and Mint, 153
Pavlova, 212–13
Peaches and "Cream" Fresh Fruit
  Smoothie, 106
pears
  Fruity Green Salad, 134
  Poached Pears, 206
  Poached Pears with Topping, 207
  Warm Poached Pear and Dried
    Fruit Compote, 208
peas, Paella, 184–85
peppers, bell, recipes for, 116–17,
  121, 126–27, 165, 179, 184–85,
  192
peppers, chile, recipes for, 121,
  126–27, 149–50, 170–71, 199
phytochemicals, 63
Pistou, 129
Pita Triangles, Toasted, 152
planning
  breakfast and, 35
  daily food, 22
  for dining out, 96–97
Poached Eggs with Veggie Hash,
  116–17
Poached Pears, 206
  with Topping, 207
Polenta with Swiss Chard and
  Portabella Mushrooms,
  168–69

polyunsaturated fats, 69, 76
Portabella Mushroom Burgers,
  156–57
potassium, 81
potatoes, 64
  Fish Chowder, 132
  Leek and Potato Soup, 125
  Lemon Parsley Chicken Breast
    with Baby Artichokes and
    Potatoes, 180
  Mashed Potatoes, 193
  Mushroom Soup, 122–23
  Oven-Baked Steak "Fries," 195
  Poached Eggs with Veggie Hash,
    116–17
  Potato Omelet, 115
  Potato Pancakes, 113
  Salade Niçoise, 145–46
  Small Rustic Roasted Red Potatoes,
    194
  Vegetable Frittata, 164
poultry, 62–63, 94
  Grilled Skinless Chicken Breasts
    with Mango-Tomato Salsa,
    181
  Lemon Parsley Chicken Breast
    with Baby Artichokes and
    Potatoes, 180
  Paella, 184–85
  Turkey Piccata, 182
  Turkey Scallopini, 183
  See also protein
praise, 14, 101
protein, 70–72
  amino acids in, 72
  calories per gram, 73
  excessive amounts of, 3, 71
  glycemic index and, 68
  percentage of total daily calories,
    71
  serving size, 62–63
  vegetable sources, 72, 80–82

protein *(cont.)*
very-low-carbohydrate, high-protein approach, 2–4, 5, 6
See also specific protein foods
Provençal Vegetable Soup *(Soupe au Pistou)*, 128–29
prunes, Warm Poached Pear and Dried Fruit Compote, 208
purslane, 70, 84

Quick Herbed Bread Crumbs, 178
quinoa, 72, 93
Quinoa Pilaf, 198

raisins, Warm Poached Pear and Dried Fruit Compote, 208
raspberries. *See* berries
Red Bean Soup, 131
Red Tomato Gazpacho, 121
refined sugar, 61, 65–66, 67, 76–78
repetitions, in strength training, 25–26
restaurants, 95–100
rewards, 14, 101, 102
rice, 93–94
Breakfast Fried Rice (With or Without Rice), 118
Hoisin Shrimp and Okra with Brown Rice, 174–75
Wild Rice Salad, 142–43
Roasted Red Beets, 189
Roasted Tomato Soup, 120

salad dressings
Light Blue Cheese, 137
Vinaigrette, 139, 140, 141, 145–46; Asparagus, 138; Citrus, 142–43; Roasted Red Pepper, 179; Walnut, 135–36
salads
Asparagus Vinaigrette, 138

Baby Greens with Warm Goat Cheese and Walnut Vinaigrette, 135–36
"convenience" packaging, 91–92
Crispy Romaine Salad with Apples, Celery, Toasted Walnuts, and Light Blue Cheese Dressing, 137
dining out, 96
Fresh Fruit Medley, 107
Fresh Summer Tomato Salad with Fresh Mozzarella and Basil, 139
Fruity Green Salad, 134
Green Bean Salad with Toasted Walnuts, 141
Healthy Coleslaw, 188
Marinated Italian Seafood Salad, 147–48
Salade Niçoise, 145–46
Summer Tomato Salad, 140
Tuna with Grape Tomatoes and Greens, 144
Wild Rice Salad, 142–43
salmon. *See* seafood and fish
salty foods, 48, 55
sandwich recipes, 154–59
saturated fatty acids, 69, 72, 76
Scarsdale diet, 3
Scrambled Egg Whites with Spinach and Orange, 114
seafood and fish, 62–63, 70, 83–84, 94–95
Artichoke and Tuna Panini, 159
Baked Lemon Herb Halibut, 176
Fish Chowder, 132
Grilled Tuna or Swordfish with Roasted Red Pepper Vinaigrette, 179
Hoisin Shrimp and Okra with Brown Rice, 174–75
Marinated Italian Seafood Salad, 147–48

Mustard-Crusted Baked Salmon, 177–78
Paella, 184–85
Pan-Seared Fillet of Tilapia with Mango Tomato Salsa and Lentil Pancake, 172–73
Salade Niçoise, 145–46
Salmon Burger, 158
Spicy Mexican Shrimp Cocktail, 149–50
Steamed Manila Clams and Mussels in White Wine Broth with Chili Flakes and Spaghetti, 170–71
Tuna with Grape Tomatoes and Greens, 144
See also protein
seeds, 72
selenium, 75, 81
serving sizes, 62–63
setbacks, 14, 100–102
sets, in strength training, 25–26
shopping, food, 84–90
shrimp. *See* seafood and fish
sleep, 15–16, 21, 22, 30, 38, 40–41, 51
Small Rustic Roasted Red Potatoes, 194
Smoothie, Peaches and "Cream" Fresh Fruit, 106
snacks
    benefits of, 53–55
    during the day, 49–50, 53–55
    before dining out, 97
    emotional eating and, 44–46, 53
    examples of, 55, 82
    late-night, 21, 22, 31, 40–49, 59
sodium, 48, 55
soft drinks, 76–77
soup recipes, 120–32, 203
soybean oils, 70, 84
soy protein, 72, 80–81
    Tofu and Broccoli Stir Fry, 162–63

sparkling water, 17
Spicy Mexican Shrimp Cocktail, 149–50
Spicy Toasted Walnuts, 217
spinach
    Scrambled Egg Whites with Spinach and Orange, 114
    Spinach Penne with Spicy Roasted Pepper Sauce, 165
Steamed Manila Clams and Mussels in White Wine Broth with Chili Flakes and Spaghetti, 170–71
Stillman diet, 2
strength training, 7–8, 9, 13–14, 24–26, 72
sugar
    blood, 30–31, 37, 51, 61, 66–68
    refined, 61, 65–66, 67, 76, 77, 78
    types of, 61, 65–66, 77–78
Summer Succotash, 192
Summer Tomato Salad, 140
supermarkets
    natural food, 87–88
    traditional, 89
supplements, 55, 56, 73–75, 77, 80–81
support, 15
Swiss chard
    Braised Swiss Chard with Raisins and Pine Nuts, 191
    Broccoli and Swiss Chard Cannelloni, 166–67
    Polenta with Swiss Chard and Portabella Mushrooms, 168–69

table sugar, 61, 65–66, 67, 76–78
target heart range, 20–21
time management, breakfast and, 34, 35
tofu, 81
    Tofu and Broccoli Stir Fry, 162–63

tomatoes
  Eggplant and Zucchini Poor Boy
    Sandwich, 154
  Fish Chowder, 132
  Fresh Summer Tomato Salad with
    Fresh Mozzarella and Basil, 139
  Grilled Skinless Chicken Breasts
    with Mango-Tomato Salsa, 181
  Marinara Sauce, 167
  Red Tomato Gazpacho, 121
  Roasted Tomato Soup, 120
  Salade Niçoise, 145–46
  Spicy Mexican Shrimp Cocktail,
    149–50
  Summer Tomato Salad, 140
  Tomatoes Stuffed with Couscous,
    Cucumber, and Mint, 153
  Tuna with Grape Tomatoes and
    Greens, 144
  Vegetable Frittata, 164
Tortilla Chips, Baked, 150
trainers, certification of, 25
trans-fatty acids, 69, 76, 82
tryptophan, 44
tuna. *See* seafood and fish
turkey. *See* poultry

Vegetable Frittata, 164
vegetables
  daily servings of, 63–64, 67
  farmers' markets and, 85–87
  glycemic index and, 67, 68
  leafy greens, 83, 91–92
  protein in, 72, 80–82

serving size, 62
  tips for buying, 90–92
  See also names of specific vegetables
vinaigrette. *See under* salad dressings
vitamins, 55, 74–75, 77
  B complex, 74–75, 81
  vitamin C, 56
  vitamin D, 75
  vitamin E, 75, 80

Warm Apple Crisp, 204–5
Warm Poached Pear and Dried Fruit
  Compote, 208
water consumption, 9, 16–18, 59
  dehydration and, 16–17, 53–55
  role in nutrition, 59–60, 76–77
water weight, 3, 71–72
weight lifting. *See* strength training
Wild Mushroom Grits, 197
Wild Rice Salad, 142–43
willpower, 14–15, 53
work habits, 42–43

Yams, Maple Glazed and Roasted,
  196
yogurt. *See* dairy products

zucchini
  Eggplant and Zucchini Poor Boy
    Sandwich, 154
  Provençal Vegetable Soup *(Soupe
    au Pistou)*, 128–29
  Zucchini with Cilantro and
    Yogurt, 190